The Juice Lady's

Guide to
FASTING

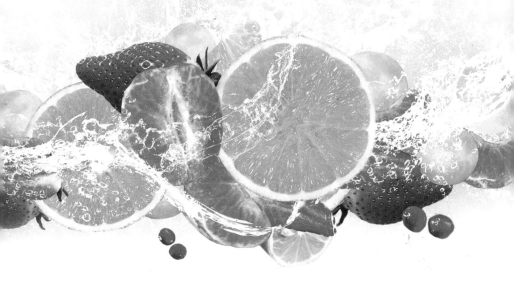

Cherie Calbom, MSN

SILOAM

Most CHARISMA HOUSE BOOK GROUP products are available at special quantity discounts for bulk purchase for sales promotions, premiums, fundraising, and educational needs. For details, write Charisma House Book Group, 600 Rinehart Road, Lake Mary, Florida 32746, or telephone (407) 333-0600.

THE JUICE LADY'S GUIDE TO FASTING by Cherie Calbom
Published by Siloam
Charisma Media/Charisma House Book Group
600 Rinehart Road
Lake Mary, Florida 32746
www.charismahouse.com

Cover design by Lisa Rae McClure
Design Director: Justin Evans

Visit the author's website at www.juiceladycherie.com.

Library of Congress Cataloging-in-Publication Data:
Names: Calbom, Cherie, author.
Title: The juice lady's guide to fasting / Cherie Calbom.
Description: Lake Mary, Florida : Siloam, [2017] | Includes bibliographical
    references.
Identifiers: LCCN 2016045379| ISBN 9781629989594 (trade paper) |
    ISBN
    9781629989600 (ebook)
Subjects: LCSH: Fasting. | Fruit juices--Therapeutic use. | Vegetable
    juices--Therapeutic use. | Fasting--Physiological aspects. |
    Fasting--Religious aspects. | Recipes.
Classification: LCC RM226.5 .C35 2017 | DDC 613.2--dc23
LC record available at https://lccn.loc.gov/2016045379

17 18 19 20 21 — 987654321
Printed in the United States of America

CONTENTS

List of Recipes... vii

Introduction..1

1 The Benefits of Fasting...9

2 The Different Fasting Diets...28

3 Water and Fasting..52

4 You Need to Detox..69

5 The Detox Fast..82

6 Frequently Asked Questions About Fasting.................115

7 The Quick and Easy Juice-Fast
   Menu and Recipes..129

8 The Daniel Fast Menu Plan..153

9 The Spirituality of Fasting...179

10 Fasting From Toxic Thinking and Emotions.................201

Appendix:
   Resources...229

Notes..234

LIST OF RECIPES

Adrenal Booster Cocktail 140

Almond Butter Balls 176

Amaranth Pumpkin Porridge 158

Anti-Inflammatory Power
    Cocktail 139

Apple Pie à la Mode 147

Arugula Spinach Blueberry
    Detox Salad 159

Asian Salad 162

Beet Salad 110

Beet-Berry Liver-Cleanse
    Cocktail 111

Beet-Berry Liver-Cleanse
    Juice 147

Blended Citrus Shake Liver-
    Gallbladder Flush 109

Blood-Sugar-Balancing
    Cocktail 142

Bone Broth 168

Broccoli Pomegranate Salad 163

Brown Lentil Rhubarb Soup 165

Burdock Root With
    Vegetables 168

Carrot and Spice 137

Carrot Cake 146

Carrot Radish Pumpkin-Seed
    Herb Salad 161

Carrot Salad With Lemon–Olive
    Oil Dressing 112

Carrot Sauce With Asparagus
    and Fresh Peas Over
    Brown Rice 173

Cherie's Awesome Green
    Smoothie 157

Chia Breakfast Pudding 154

Cholesterol-Lowering Juice
    Cocktail 144

Cider-Braised Greens and
    Green Beans 171

Cilantro Heavy-Metal-Detox
    Cocktail 143

Colon-Flush Juice Cocktail 106

Creamy Basil-Cumin-Carrot
    Soup 150

Creamy Carrot-Ginger-Lime
    Soup 150

Creamy Green Smoothie
    Bowl 149

Creamy Spinach Soup 151

Creamy Zucchini Soup With
    Chopped Almonds 151

Curb-Your-Carb-Cravings
    Juice 143

Dandelion-Coconut Water 136

Dehydrated Zucchini Chips 176

DIY Fiber Blend 108

DIY Salad With Avocado and
    Chickpeas With Lemon-
    Tarragon Dressing 162

Donna's Zucchini Salad 160

Easy Lentil Skillet Dinner 174

Fabulous Gluten-Free
    Pancakes 155

Fat Flush Ambrosia 139

Fiber Shake 108

Fire and Ice 140

Garlic Love Weight Loss
    Cocktail 142

Get Your Ginger Greens On 138

Ginger Limeade 146

Green Drink 111

Green Muscle Mender 146

Green Power Morning 135

Happy-Mood Morning.................136
Herb and Chickpea
Croquettes.................170
Herb and Chickpea Croquettes
With Rosemary-Walnut Pesto,
and Cider-Braised Greens and
Green Beans.................170
Immune Booster Shot.................138
Kale Chips.................175
Kidney Tonic Juice.................114
Kidney-Cleansing Cocktail.................145
Lemon-Herb White-Bean Soup.....167
Lemon-Tahini Sauce
(or Dressing).................169
Lemon-Tarragon Vinaigrette.........163
Liver Detox Juice Cocktail.................141
Liver-Cleansing Cocktail.................110
Metabolism Booster Juice.................140
Nettle Tea.................114
Nut-and-Seed Morning
Smoothie.................156
Onion Rings.................175
Overnight Soaked Muesli.................157
Pink Ginger Lady.................148
Prickly Pink.................145
Pumpkin Curry Soup.................166
Quinoa With White Beans and
Roasted Peppers.................171
Red Cabbage-Jicama-Carrot-
Lime Cocktail.................134
Red Sunrise.................133
Refreshing Mint Cooler.................136
Refreshing Rejuvenator.................141
Revitalizing Tomato-Coconut
Juice.................134
Rosemary-Walnut Pesto.................171

Rosy Glow.................133, 146
Saltwater Flush.................39
Sesame Kale Salad With
Apple.................161
Shamrock Green Detox
Shake.................149
Skinny-Sip Sparkling
Lemonade.................144
Snappy Water.................63
South-of-the-Border Lettuce
Wraps.................172
Spiced Eggplant and Sweet
Potato Stew.................166
Spicy Lentil Soup With Delicata
Squash.................164
Spicy Veggie.................145
Sprouted Buckwheat Cereal.......156
Squash and Arugula
Enchiladas.................173
Strawberry-Kale Smoothie
Supreme.................148
Sun Water.................63
Sweet Potato–Black Bean–
Quinoa Burgers With Lemon-
Tahini Sauce.................169
The Feel Good Cocktail.................141
The Ginger Hopper With
a Twist.................138
Tomato Florentine With
a Twist.................135
Vegan Cheese.................176
Very Veggie Green-Bean
Soup.................164
Wheatgrass Juice
Pick-Me-Up.................107
Wild Greens Detox Juice.............111, 144

INTRODUCTION

N O STRANGER TO fasting, I've embarked on nearly every fasting diet in this book. They all have benefits, but nothing has offered better results for me than juice fasting. My juicing and fasting journey started years before I became "the Juice Lady." But it was a serendipitous request from the owners of the Juiceman company that led to my becoming known as the Juice Lady on TV and in print. I was living in Seattle, Washington, completing graduate school at Bastyr University (a school of naturopathic medicine), when another graduate student and I were asked to write a booklet containing juice recipes and nutrition information to accompany the Juiceman Juicer. One thing led to another, and before long I was traveling around the country almost weekly as the Juice Lady, teaching people how to create nutritious juices that are guaranteed to renew health and vitality.

Even before I decided to pursue my master's degree in whole-foods nutrition science, I had a passionate personal interest in the benefits of high-quality nutrition because it was juicing, detoxing, fasting, and eating whole organic foods that had brought me back to full health not just once, but twice. Now I want nothing more than to bring other people along with me on the journey to a life of health and wholeness.

In this book I want to introduce you to the unlimited benefits of fasting to help you prevent disease, heal your body, lose weight, and improve your health on all levels—body, soul, and spirit. As I'm writing this introduction, I'm fasting today. I just drank my gazpacho in a glass. It's delicious and satisfying. But I've realized again just how often I want to eat something out of habit or diversion from my work. It's the only time I allow myself a break when I'm writing. Well, I didn't have that excuse today. I wasn't overly hungry, but I felt emotionally deprived. I was reminded firsthand about the struggles and temptations that come with fasting. Nevertheless, I have forged ahead. I know you can too.

JUICING AND FASTING CHANGED MY LIFE

Years ago I discovered the healing power of freshly made juice as well as raw foods, whole foods, and yes, juice fasting. I'd like to share my story with you.

Sick and tired of being sick and tired

I had been sick for a few years and just kept getting worse. I was so sick and tired, I could barely walk around the house. I wondered, "Will I ever be well again?" I'd had to quit my job when I turned thirty because I had chronic fatigue syndrome and fibromyalgia. They made me so sick I couldn't work. I felt as though I had a never-ending flu. Constantly feverish with swollen glands and perennial lethargy, I was also in constant pain. My body ached all over.

I had moved back to my father's home in Colorado to try to recover. But not one doctor had a recommendation for what I should do to facilitate healing. So I went to some health-food stores and browsed around, talked with employees, and read a few books. I decided that everything I'd been doing—eating fast food, having granola for dinner, and not eating vegetables—was tearing down my health rather than healing my body. I read about juicing and whole foods, and it made sense to me. So I bought a juicer and designed a program I could follow.

I kicked off my new program with a five-day juice fast. On the fifth day my body expelled a tumor the size of a golf ball with blue blood vessels attached. I was surprised and actually encouraged. I thought I'd be well in short order.

But that was not to be the case.

I continued juicing and ate a nearly perfect diet of live and whole foods for three months. There were ups and downs throughout. I had days on which I felt encouraged that I was making some progress but other days on which I felt worse. The latter were discouraging and made me wonder if health was my elusive dream. No one told me about detox reactions, which was what I was experiencing. I was obviously very toxic, and my body was cleansing away all that stuff that had made me sick. This caused the not-so-good days in the midst of the promising ones.

But one morning I woke up early—early for me, which was around 8:00 a.m.—without an alarm sounding off. I felt as if someone had given me a new body in the night. I had so much energy, I actually wanted to go jogging! What had happened? This new sensation of health seemed to have appeared with the morning sun. But actually my body had been healing all along; the healing simply had not manifested until that day.

What a wonderful sense of being alive! I looked and felt completely renewed. With my juicer in tow and a new lifestyle fully embraced, I returned to Southern California a few weeks later to finish writing my first book. For nearly a year I enjoyed great health and more energy and stamina than I'd ever remembered.

But just ahead was a shattering event.

Death came calling

The Fourth of July was a beautiful day like so many others in Southern California. I celebrated the holiday with friends that evening at a backyard barbecue. When the evening got cool, we put on jackets and watched fireworks light up the night sky. I had been house-sitting for some vacationing friends who lived in a lovely neighborhood nearby, and I returned just before midnight. Soon I was snug in bed.

I woke up shivering sometime later. "Why is it so cold?" I wondered as I rolled over to see the clock. It was 3:00 a.m.

That's when I noticed that the door to the backyard was open. "Wonder how that happened?" I thought as I began to get up to close and lock it. Suddenly I noticed a young man crouched in the shadows of the corner of the room—a shirtless guy in shorts. I blinked twice, trying to deny what I was seeing.

Instead of running away, he leaped off the floor and ran toward me. He pulled a pipe from his shorts and began attacking me, beating me repeatedly over the head and yelling, "Now you are dead!"

We fought—or, I should say, I tried to defend myself and grab the pipe. It finally flew out of his hands. That's when he choked me to unconsciousness.

I felt life leaving my body. "This is it—the end of my life," I thought. I felt sad for the people who loved me and about how they would feel about this tragic event. Then I felt my spirit leave in a sensation of popping out of my body and floating upward. Suddenly everything was peaceful and still. I sensed I was traveling at what seemed like the speed of light through black space. I saw what looked like lights twinkling in the distance.

But all of a sudden I was back in my body, outside the house, clinging to a fence at the end of the dog run. I don't know how I got there. I screamed for help with all the breath I had. My third scream took all my strength. I felt it would be my last. Each time I screamed, I passed out and landed on the cement. I then had to pull myself up again. But this time a neighbor heard me and sent her husband to help. Within a short time I was on my way to the hospital.

Lying on a cold gurney at 4:30 a.m., chilled to the bone, in and out of consciousness, I tried to assess my injuries. When I finally looked at my right hand, I almost passed out again. My ring finger was barely hanging on by a small piece of skin. My hand was split open, and I could see deep inside.

The next thing I knew, I was being wheeled off to surgery. Later I learned that I had suffered serious injuries to my head, neck, back, and right hand, with multiple head wounds and part of my scalp torn from my head. I also incurred numerous cracked teeth that required several root canals and crowns months later.

My right hand sustained the most severe injuries, with two knuckles crushed to mere bone fragments and powder that had to be held together by three metal pins. Six months after the attack I still couldn't use it. The cast I wore—with bands holding up the ring finger, plus various odd-shaped molded parts—looked like something from a science-fiction movie. I felt and looked worse than hopeless, with a shaved top of my head, totally red and swollen eyes, a gash on my face, a useless right hand, an ongoing terrorizing fear, and barely enough energy to get dressed in the morning. I was an emotional wreck.

I couldn't sleep at night—not even a minute. It was torturous. Never mind that I was staying with a cousin and his family. There was no need to worry about safety from a practical point of view, but that made no difference emotionally. I'd lie in bed all night and stare at the ceiling or the bedroom door. I had five lights that I kept on all night. I'd try to read, but my eyes would sting. I could sleep for only a little while during the day.

But the worst part was the pain in my soul that nearly took my breath away. All the emotional pain of the attack combined with the pain and trauma of my past felt like an emotional tsunami. My past had been riddled with loss, trauma, and anxiety. My brother had died when I was two. My mother had died of cancer when I was six. I couldn't remember much about her death—the memories seemed blocked. But my cousin said I fainted at her funeral. That told me the impact was huge. I had lived for the next three years with my father and maternal grandparents. But Grandpa John died when I was nine. The loss was immeasurable. Four years later my father was involved in a very tragic situation that would take far too long to discuss here. He was no longer in my daily life. I felt terrified about my future. My grandmother was eighty-six. I had no idea how many more years she would live. The next year I moved to Oregon to live with an aunt and uncle until I graduated from high school.

Wrapped in my soul was a big package of anguish and pain with all sorts of triggers. To heal physically, mentally, and emotionally after the attack took every ounce of my will, faith, and trust in God. I did deep spiritual work, sought alternative medical help, took extra vitamins and minerals, resumed vegetable juicing, and experienced the emotional release of healing prayer and numerous detox programs.

I met a nutritionally minded physician who had healed his own slow-mending broken bones with lots of vitamin-mineral IVs. He gave me similar IVs. Juicing, cleansing, fasting, nutritional supplements, a nearly perfect diet, prayer, and physical therapy helped my bones and other injuries heal.

After I followed this regimen for about nine months, what my hand surgeon said was impossible became a reality—a fully restored, fully functional hand. He had told me it wasn't possible to put in plastic knuckles because of the hand's poor condition and that I'd never use my right hand again. But my knuckles did indeed re-form—primarily due to prayer—and the function of my hand returned. A day came when he told me I was completely healed, and though he admitted he didn't believe in miracles, he said, "You're the closest thing I've seen to one."

The healing of my hand was indeed a miracle! I had a useful hand again, and my career in writing was not over, as I had thought it would be.

My inner wounds were more severe than the physical devastation, however, and they were the hardest to heal. Nevertheless, they mended too. I experienced healing from the painful memories and trauma of the attack and the wounds from the past through prayer, letting go, forgiveness, laying on of hands, and deep emotional healing work. I called the ladies "angels" who prayed for me around their kitchen tables week after week until my soul was healed. I cried endless buckets of tears that had been pent up in my soul. I desperately needed the release. Forgiveness and letting go came in stages and proved to be an integral part of my total healing. I had to be honest about what I really felt and to be willing to face the pain and toxic emotions confined inside and then let them go.

Finally, after a very long journey, I felt free. Eventually I could even celebrate the Fourth of July without fear. Today I know more peace and health than I ever thought would be possible. I have experienced what it is to feel whole and complete—not damaged, broken, wounded, or impaired. I feel safe in the world, truly healed and restored in body, soul, and spirit.

I have learned that my purpose is to love you to life through my writing and nutritional information and to help you find the way to wholeness. If I could recover from all that had happened to me, you can too. Even if you have an illness or face frustration at not being able to lose the weight you want, I want to encourage you that you can do this.

You can fast and experience the amazing benefits. No matter what you face, there is hope. I want you to know that I think you are awesome for buying a book on fasting. I cheer you on as you fast from many foods you like and from the thoughts and emotions that clog your soul.

I tell my story here because I refer to it in other parts of the book, especially in the chapter on emotional and mental fasting. It's been an incredible journey for me of letting go of (fasting from) negative thoughts and emotions to facilitate the healing of my soul. That was difficult. But fasting from food is something I thought I could never do because of having hypoglycemia (low blood sugar). Yet vegetable juice fasting brought a great deal of healing to my body, and I was happy to be able to do something I didn't think was possible for me.

I've seen fasting change the lives and health of many people I've worked with. I shared my story of the burglar attack with you as an example of what emotional and mental fasting can do to bring hope and healing to your soul, which also greatly impacts your body. In the end I found it more difficult to fast from toxic thoughts and emotions than to fast from food. Letting go of fear was the struggle of my life. But if I had not been able to let go of fear, anger, resentment, and bitterness, I would not be here today, leading the way for others—including you—to find help and healing too.

Vision of Insight

Years ago I had a vision of soldiers lying on a battlefield with their armor askew. They were in pain, and written in banners across their bodies were names of diseases, such as cancer, heart disease, diabetes, chronic fatigue, lupus, MS, arthritis…on and on it went. I saw people with cold packs on their heads and holding various parts of their bodies that were in pain. I heard a voice saying, "These people are sick because they don't know how to care for their bodies. Teach them how to eat and how to live."

Shortly after that vision I went back to graduate school and completed my degree in whole-foods nutrition from Bastyr University. I've been teaching people what they can do to heal ever since that time.

Fasting is a big part of the healing process. You'll see in the next chapter all the scientific evidence of what fasting can do to heal the body.

Though I fast regularly at certain times of the year, I also live a fasted lifestyle. I fast two days a week. I never eat sweets; sugar is not a part of my life in any way, shape, or form, not even on special occasions. I don't eat gluten, dairy, or junk food, and I rarely eat anything but organic food. I don't drink coffee, except for an occasional unsweetened almond-milk latte. Fast food is not something I order when I'm out and about. I don't drink alcohol—ever. This is my life, my path of freedom and health. It's had huge payoffs for me.

I also have chosen to fast from negative thoughts and emotions. When people do things that are offensive, I seek ways to turn the situation around and defuse an emotional charge. It's taken me years to learn this lesson and to choose to live from a positive attitude. I know you can find this path too. That doesn't mean we need to be pushovers. Far from it. But we can remain strong and positive.

I hope and pray that you will glean many benefits from fasting. I encourage you to try a variety of fasts in this book. I also encourage you to read the chapter on the spirituality of fasting. We are living at a time in history when fasting and prayer are vitally important for us and for our nation. We can't afford *not* to fast.

Emotional and mental fasting also are needed. This type of fasting is as important as any food fast. We've seen the power of it at our juice and raw-foods fasting retreats. As people fast, many emotions bubble up that were regularly stuffed down with food. As toxic emotions are let go, healing is experienced.

There's a purpose for your life, just as there is for mine. You need to be strong and well to complete your purpose. You can be greatly served by a positive mind and an optimistic attitude along with a strong, healthy body. You can fast for breakthroughs physically, spiritually, emotionally, and financially. With God's help and the latest information on fasting provided in this book, you can facilitate abundant health, learn the right way to live your life to the fullest, and finish well.

Chapter 1

THE BENEFITS OF FASTING

I fast for greater physical and mental efficiency.
—PLATO

'M SO GLAD you are interested in the practice of fasting. The benefits are endless and include the healing of ailments, stem-cell regeneration, weight loss, the curing of food addictions, spiritual renewal, and revival of soul. What do you hope to achieve with your fast? I recommend you list the reasons you want to fast before beginning. And whatever you list, get ready—you may get far more from your fast than you ever hoped!

According to multiple news reports, fasting is gaining in popularity. Perhaps its emerging popularity is our cultural way of responding to a nation gone wild on a food binge: "The number of obese Americans is now greater than the number who are merely overweight, according to government figures released in January [2009]."[1]

Though newly popular in our times, fasting itself is not new. Plato, Socrates, Aristotle, Galen, and other early philosophers, thinkers, and healers praised the benefits of fasting and used it for health and as a healing therapy. Paracelsus, a father of Western medicine, said, "Fasting is the greatest remedy—the physician within."[2] Plato said he used fasting to increase his physical and mental efficiency.

Even students of early healing arts dating back to Hippocrates (460–370 BC) knew the revitalizing and rejuvenating power found in regular fasting. As the father of modern medicine, Hippocrates prescribed fasting and drinking apple cider vinegar as part of his healing treatments and protocols. He has been quoted as saying, "To eat when you are sick, is to feed your illness."[3] Greek historian and writer Plutarch shared these views and wrote, "Instead of using medicine, better fast today."[4] Benjamin Franklin, one of America's Founding Fathers, said, "The best of all medicines is resting and fasting."[5]

Almost every major religion in the world includes fasting as part of its spiritual or health practice. From Christianity, Judaism, and Islam to Buddhism, Hinduism, and American Indian traditions, world religions tap into the benefits of fasting for "purification, spiritual vision, penance, mourning, sacrifice," and even "to prevent or break the habits of gluttony."[6] Orthodox Christians, Roman Catholics, Anglicans, Lutherans, and Jews are the most well known for continuing fasting practices in the United States today.[7]

You've heard the benefits of following the Mediterranean diet. Studies of people in cities such as those on the Greek island of Crete support these claims. But what Dr. Ancel Keys, the American scientist who introduced the Mediterranean diet, may have missed is that the amazing health he observed in the people of Crete was partly due to their adherence to the Greek Orthodox tradition of fasting.[8] A friend of ours told my husband and me about eating at a Greek restaurant where one of the owners served him. He learned that she was actually the grandmother of the family and was in her seventies. He said she looked like a vibrant woman not much over fifty—not much older than her daughter. When he asked her about her secret, she said, "I'm Greek Orthodox, and I attribute it to all the fasting we do."

In the early 1900s Linda Hazzard wrote *Fasting for the Cure of Disease*. Based on her training as a nurse, the content of the book supports her claim that eating only a small amount of food could cure diseases such as cancer. Though one of her patients died of starvation— and Hazzard went to prison because of it—health experts are resurrecting some of her conclusions regarding how restricted eating could aid people with cancer and other illnesses.[9]

In a study on fasting, Valter Longo, director of the University of Southern California's Longevity Institute, determined that when fasting two to five days each month, mice showed "reduced biomarkers for diabetes, cancer, and heart disease. The research has since been expanded to people, and scientists saw a similar reduction in disease risk factors."[10] The study revealed another benefit of fasting: it helps lower insulin levels and "another hormone called insulin such as growth factor, or IGF-1, which is linked to cancer and diabetes."[11] Longo says that when you fast, your cells enter a "protected mode."[12]

Expanding his research to humans, Dr. Longo's team led a group of nineteen healthy adults through three three-month cycles during which they ate a plant-based diet consisting of "34% and 54% of the normal caloric intake with at least 9–10% protein, 34–47% carbohydrate, and 44–56% fat" for five days out of each of the three months.[13] During the rest of each month they ate their usual diet. Another group of nineteen adults maintained their regular eating habits all days of the three-month cycles. The nineteen who followed the researchers' prescribed diet noted "improvements in blood glucose and decreased body weight" as compared with the group of adults who maintained their usual diets.[14] The individuals who started the study with higher C-reactive protein levels (a protein that indicates risk levels for heart disease) ended the program with lower levels. Those who had normal levels did not experience any change. Though side effects were minimal, some participants felt tired and weak. Some experienced headaches.

Longo commented on the reasoning behind the diet he used during his study: "Strict fasting is hard for people to stick to, and it can also be dangerous, so we developed a complex diet that triggers the same effects in the body. It's not a typical diet because it isn't something you need to stay on."[15]

In light of the long-standing history of fasting and current research that supports what people have known for centuries, it's safe to say it has proven benefits. This time-honored tradition is actually an ancient treasure that's gaining new respect in the modern world.

THE SKINNY ON FASTING

Fasting is an ancient tradition of abstaining from food and/or drink. According to the dictionary, to *fast* means to "eat sparingly or abstain from some foods" for a period of time.[16] A fast also may be intermittent in time.

There are many ways to fast, but often people think of water-only fasts when they consider fasting. They don't realize you can abstain for a period of time from anything you would normally eat or drink, and that's considered fasting. A strict water fast is so severe that many people feel there is no way they could ever take on such a feat. Jennifer Eivaz, in her article for *Charisma News*, says:

> I love the idea of going on an extended fast, but I'm pretty sure that I will die if I do! Fasting is something I struggle with. I just happen to be one of those kind, loving individuals who turns into a monster if they do not eat regularly. Hopefully you hear my humor in that statement, but to a certain extent, it's true. People with a sensitive physiology and low-blood sugar problems can take on a certain form of crazy when they haven't eaten on time.[17]

I'm here to tell you that you can fast *and* eat! If you want to embark on a fast for physical and/or spiritual reasons, there's a long history of fasting during Lent and many other periods throughout the year when people eat food—vegan food. Some people call this the Daniel fast. There are other fasts, such as a juice fast or a liquid diet that includes smoothies. You have many options besides the strict water fast that won't send your blood sugar into the basement along with your blood pressure. With these fasts you still can facilitate a spiritual and physical transformation.

THE CURATIVE POWER OF FASTING

When we're not eating food throughout the day, we free up our digestive system from a lot of its work, so the body can refocus its energies on cleansing, healing, repairing, restoring, and regenerating. Our bodies are made to heal themselves, but we must provide the right environment for that to happen. Fasting provides that environment. During a fast, dead cells, cysts, tumors, pockets of toxins, and other irritants that cause disease can be broken down and moved out of the body. Such things as dissolving calcium deposits in the joints; releasing toxins stored in the liver, kidneys, muscles, and fat cells; repairing scar tissue; and restoring or removing aging, injured, or infected cells all can happen when the body is not burdened with the many processes involved in our digestion of food. Also, the raw juices consumed during juice fasts provide our bodies with much-needed enzymes that the body does not need to manufacture itself as part of the normal digestive process, allowing it to focus more attention on other areas of need.

The rate at which our bodies heal during a fast is simply amazing. You wouldn't believe how many health issues just go away. During one of my juice fasts a mole on my arm just fell off! My sinuses totally cleared up during a liver flush. If you have skin irritations or achy joints and muscles, you may be surprised how quickly you find relief during a fast. You may even notice that skin issues clear up—a skin tag may disappear, or a dark patch of skin may go away.[18]

My experience with fasting is that it can heal even more serious health issues such as chronic fatigue syndrome and fibromyalgia. As I mentioned in the introduction, many years ago when I was very sick, I started my healing journey with a five-day juice fast, and on day five my body expelled a tumor the size of a golf ball with blue blood vessels attached. I was totally amazed that a juice fast could produce that kind of result! Years later, when I was working on my master's thesis titled "Nutrition and Cancer," I found research indicating that glutathione, a tripeptide, and certain flavonoids—all found in fruits and vegetables—can cut off the blood supply to tumors. It seems as if this is what happened in my body that caused me to expel the tumor.

Research provides the following support for this theory:

> When human blood vessel cells are stimulated, they begin forming tubular structures. These structures develop into new capillaries, providing a blood supply to the new tumor. However, when plant flavones were added, like "apigen" or "luteolin," tube formation was blocked. These flavones are found in foods such as citrus, celery, peppers, and throughout the plant kingdom. Similarly, "fisitin" which is found in strawberries and many other fruits and

vegetables, also significantly shrank the formation of new blood vessels.[19]

Peter Seewald in *Wisdom From the Monastery* says, "In many cases it [fasting] works like an 'operation without a knife.' No surgeon's scalpel can remove what is harmful to the body as carefully, skillfully, and painlessly, while preserving what is useful, as the fasting body itself."[20]

Due to increased interest in fasting, researchers have embarked upon a new series of studies and have found that fasting can benefit people with cancer, Alzheimer's, Parkinson's, and dementia. It also has been shown to help "guard against diabetes and heart disease, [and] help control asthma."[21]

Most research on how eating habits affect health and longevity deals mainly with calorie restriction and boasts some pretty outstanding outcomes. Still, fasting entirely from food on certain days of the week, month, or year "brings about biochemical and physiological changes that daily dieting does not."[22]

Some experts who study the eating habits of early humans believe that we are naturally made to go without food periodically. Mark Mattson, a diet researcher at the National Institute on Aging, says that "the evidence is pretty strong that our ancestors did not eat three meals a day plus snacks. Our genes are geared to being able to cope with periods of no food."[23]

One concern with calorie restriction is that some people could become more susceptible to infections and biological stress. But with fasting, these symptoms are virtually nonexistent. The late Dr. Herbert Shelton, a natural hygienist who had a Texas-based fasting retreat and health school, said:

> Only through rest can the enervated body muster sufficient nerve energy with which to increase its work of elimination. By physiological rest is meant fasting.... Once fasting and rest have enabled the body to eliminate its stored up toxins and recuperate its nerve energy, a physiological mode of living will enable the patient to

grow into better and better health until full health is reached, and to maintain health thereafter.[24]

My Pain Is Gone!

"I'm so excited! After years of being in constant pain, doing the juice fasting and colon cleanse has alleviated a good portion of the pain. Thanks for being such a great leader and health advocate. Cheers to you!" —Karen

Dr. Alan Goldhamer says:

> During the past seven years I've worked with thousands of patients from all over the world who had a wide variety of disorders and health concerns. A great many of these patients required a period of supervised fasting to achieve their health goals. Virtually all of them needed to make lifestyle changes to achieve improved health. Fasting made the transition easier!...
>
> Fasting, for as few as five days to as many as 40 days, will often dramatically shorten the time it takes for an individual to make the transition from a conventional diet and lifestyle (with all the associated addictions, pains, fatigue and disease) to the independent and energetic state associated with healthful living.
>
> People who undertake a fast in a supervised setting tend to achieve health more quickly than those who attempt changes without a fast.[25]

Juice fasting has been shown to be the fastest way to reverse the symptoms and effects of rheumatoid arthritis (RA). When followed by a vegetarian diet, juice fasting produced substantial long-term results in a study of twenty-seven RA patients. For four weeks researchers monitored the patients during their stay at a health care facility. Even a year later those who maintained a vegetarian diet still showed marked changes in their health.[26]

Fasting Heals . . .

- Arteriosclerosis
- Asthma
- Cancer
- Chronic inflammation
- Constipation
- Glaucoma
- Gout
- Heart disorders
- High blood pressure
- Infections

- Migraine headaches
- Poor circulation
- Receding gums
- Rheumatoid arthritis
- Skin problems
- Stomach and digestive problems
- Type 2 diabetes
- Varicose veins

(Note: This list is not exhaustive. Fasting has helped almost every ailment known to mankind.)[27]

Better than any herb, vitamin, or natural supplement, juice fasting also provides healing benefits for acute conditions such as the flu, colds, bronchial infections, kidney stones, and more. When combined with herbal teas and tinctures, juice fasts with fresh raw juice are the quickest route to healing.

YOU REALLY CAN LOSE FIVE POUNDS IN A WEEK

At our juice-and-raw-foods retreats we typically see people lose between five and ten pounds in a week. By flushing out toxins and returning the body to its rightful balance, fasting offers unique weight-loss benefits not offered by a typical diet. Curious? Well, here's how it works.

I said earlier that fasting frees up the energy your body normally would use in digestion to focus on other duties, such as removing toxins out of fat cells. As this happens, your body can then let go of the fat cells because it is being flooded with antioxidants that help bind up the toxins and carry them away. In addition, the abundance of enzymes you consume in the raw juice breaks down protein, fat, and carbs more efficiently, giving the enzyme-producing organs a break. Mucus and pockets of toxins such as those found in cellulite are broken up, and your body can now cleanse the lymphatic system, lungs, skin, blood, kidneys, and bladder.

It's like a full makeover for your metabolism! Depending on how long you fast, you could see significant weight loss and healing.

Amazing—Six Pounds Gone in a Week!

"Thanks again for a wonderful retreat. I lost six pounds and haven't put it back on yet, so YAY! I'm juicing at least once a day." —Julie

Give your HGH a boost

Human growth hormone (HGH) plays a significant role in weight loss because of how it boosts metabolism by increasing fat burning and utilizing protein (sparing the body's process of pulling energy from other sources, such as fatty tissue, dietary fats, and carbohydrates, instead of from protein). You can see how this might help you lose weight. HGH also improves brain function and neuron processing; strengthens muscles, tendons, ligaments, and bones; and enhances the appearance and function of the skin.[28]

After fasting for twenty-four hours, a group of men and women were tested for HGH levels at the Intermountain Medical Center Heart Institute. HGH levels in the men increased by 2,000 percent, and there was a 1,300 percent increase in the women. Reduced triglycerides, increased good HDL cholesterol, and stabilized blood sugar were among the other health improvements experienced by study participants.[29] It is important, though, to find the right balance between insulin and HGH. HGH repairs tissue, fuels the body efficiently, and manages anti-inflammatory immune activity, while insulin manages energy storage, divides cells, and activates pro-inflammatory immunity. Researchers have discovered that these substances are on opposite sides of the body's metabolic processes.[30] Insulin comes into play when you eat carbohydrates, but HGH is inhibited at this stage. It also is inhibited if you consume too much protein or fat.

Fasting decreases insulin levels in the body. Metabolic problems can occur with increased insulin levels. But times of fasting bring balance to the body. They are also good for the brain; in fact, they are "essential for the brain to clean itself up and drive new neurons and communication lines for optimal function."[31]

Fasting and Fat

Fasting is also a great tool to help curb cravings and the emotional eating that often accompanies obesity or being overweight. Additionally it helps detox and cleanse the liver and gallbladder and balances hormones.

As crazy as the possibility may seem, it is actually important to avoid over-consuming calories while on a juice fast. Stick with juicing low-sugar fruit, such as green apples and berries, just to sweeten the vegetable-juice combinations. And as you begin to incorporate solid food after your fast, do not return to refined, processed, high-calorie foods. I recommend that you follow the dietary guidelines in my book *The Juice Lady's Anti-Inflammation Diet* to maintain your restored health and new weight.

Concerning weight loss, I will say first that you are made up of many patterns, beliefs, memories, and life experiences, and because of this, your journey to a healthy weight is personal and unique. Your body is also distinctly special, like a bouquet of flowers. There is not another body out there quite like yours. What makes fasting such a great discipline for anyone to add to his lifestyle habits is this: it brings healing to the various facets of your unique being on many levels and in a variety of ways. If you're fasting to lose weight, you're in for a wonderful surprise because there are so many other benefits you receive as you fast. For example, check out chapters 9 and 10 on the spirituality of fasting and fasting emotionally and mentally.

We often limit our weight-loss journey to the foods we eat, employing a strict diet—and in some cases a fad diet—that doesn't address the deeper issues contributing to our being overweight or obese. It is not always about food alone. What you hear from people who have lost weight and gone on to keep it off is the revelation they gained about the attitudes, beliefs, and emotions that had contributed to their weight gain. They also testify to the roadblocks they had to overcome in order to let go of those damaging beliefs, exchanging them for ones that support their healthy lifestyle goals. Health is not just about the number on the scale. It is also about becoming a fully vibrant and balanced healthy person—mind, body, and spirit. Those who have succeeded in shedding pounds speak of having developed a mind-set that enables them to maintain a healthy weight permanently.

If you've taken the time to evaluate your own process when it comes to weight loss, you already may have realized that your struggle has very little to do with the food you eat. You may have come to terms with past experiences or issues that relate to love, value, self-esteem, a desire for peace and harmony, and any number of other concerns. We all have them. What you will find as you join me on this journey is that fasting has a way of reaching deep into these places, especially as you combine the spiritual and emotional fasting we discuss later in the book with the dietary fasting protocols I'll guide you to try throughout the book.

Your journey is about more than just the scale. It is about your whole, beautiful self finding exceptional health at every level.

WHAT ARE YOU REALLY CRAVING?

Sometimes when we think we are hungry for food, we actually may be dehydrated. (See chapter 3 for more on this truth.) But on a deeper level we may be craving fulfillment and satisfaction in an area of our lives that seems out of our reach. Often we're seeking love, understanding, and acceptance of who we are. We're hoping to latch on to a source of fulfillment, power, and purpose greater than ourselves. Instead of discovering our genuine need and filling it, we reach for food. At times we eat and eat and still feel empty because we are craving something emotional or spiritual rather than food but don't realize it.

Fasting exposes these areas because during a fast, food cannot be used to fill the emotional or spiritual needs as they arise. It cannot stuff down the pain or anguish rising up from past experiences. We end up having to bravely face and address it instead of covering it up with food. In his book *Wisdom From the Monastery* Peter Seewald says, "Through fasting one lets go of all of the desires and needs that might obstruct one's vision."[32]

When you fast, you have a chance to see more clearly what may be holding you back from living the healthy life you desire. "Profound changes take place," says Dr. Allan Cott, author of *Fasting: The Ultimate Diet.* "These changes revise attitudes about food and put appetite into alignment with the body's real needs for energy."[33] And because of what it can reveal about us, fasting provides us with better chances to permanently manage our weight than any diet, even after the period of fasting has ended.

Fasting has a way of opening a door into the world that has the gifts we're seeking and the God who put those yearnings there in the first place. It is no wonder many of us feel lost and without peace and purpose. But in the silent space of a fast we are able to focus in and listen to our whole being and hear what life plans—spiritual, emotional, and physical—the Creator has for us.

We live in a busy, noisy world in which people expect everything to continually become bigger, faster, better. The more we have to do, the more important and valuable we seem. Even our food is highly stimulating to keep us moving on the fast track—salt, sugar, and flavor-enhancers hook us, making us want more and more. We are constantly overstimulated, overwhelmed, and over-consumed. Here's where fasting makes its heroic entrance.

Amidst all the hustle and bustle, both inside and outside our bodies, fasting cuts out all the stimulation of food and moves us into a place of quiet, giving us extra time to listen within. During a fast you cannot continue at the same pace. Because you aren't eating solid foods—or, as with a Daniel fast, you aren't eating animal foods—and have decreased your caloric intake, you have to slow your body down. It is in this place of stillness and rest where many distractions are put on pause and you are able to listen more easily for revelation on what you need to let go of, hold on to, and pick up to carry with you into the next healthier season of life. Without the stimulation of food your body becomes quieter and more at peace. You can focus on things of real value, identify destructive patterns in your life, and begin to experience more fully the blessings and guidance of God.

As you move through the chapters of this book, you will uncover ways you can receive fully the benefits of fasting, and you will see that food is only one part of the experience. Decreasing the influence of the outside world and increasing your connection to your inner world are essential practices during a fast that allow you to tune in to the subtle whispers of your heart, soul (mind, will, and emotions), and body, answering them with exactly what they need. No cover-ups—emotional eating, workaholism, sugar or caffeine addiction, or even drug addiction—allowed.

Because the diversions are diminished, fasting intensifies the connection between you and God and you and yourself, leading to the ultimate healing of your metabolism, your body, and your soul. Encouraging change in thinking patterns and core beliefs, fasting simultaneously will transform you on the inside and change you on the outside. You will eliminate toxins and waste, giving your body a chance to heal. You will not only look slimmer; you will also look more vibrant. What hot diet trend can give you all this?

Down Fifteen Pounds in Thirty Days

"I just wanted to say thank you for thirty great days [on the Thirty-Day Detox Challenge]. The juices [and three-day juice fast] were awesome. I lost fifteen pounds. Thank you." —Lana

NOT FAST ENOUGH: ANTIAGING AND A YOUNGER YOU

It has yet to be explained why fasting—and especially juice fasting—works such a miracle in our bodies, but *miracle* is the right word. The visible benefits it provides are outstanding, including a reduction in the number and depth of facial lines; an improvement in the skin's texture, firmness, and contour; and a vibrant, healthy glow to the skin, eyes, and hair. People report that even their cellulite is gone. The reason fresh juices, which I incorporate into most of the fasting protocols, are able to transform one's appearance echoes similar theories that are offered about how to slow the aging process.

At the cellular level, aging is brought about by free-radical damage to cells and an accumulation of wastes and toxins. Waste builds up because of environmental toxins, stress, and poor eating habits, which impair cellular metabolism and gradually poison and age the body. Juice fasts (or incorporating juicing with other types of fasts), which consist of drinking mainly freshly made vegetable juice with a little fruit juice for flavor for several days, are believed to counteract waste buildup by flushing away internal sludge. When you embark on a fast, you give your digestive tract a rest and enable immune cells to destroy dead, diseased, and damaged cells. At the same time the rich concentration of nutrients from the juices helps renew your cells.

Researchers have found that sparse eating, which is a part of inter-mittent fasting (fasting two days a week on a low-calorie diet), combined with longer periods of fasting slows down the rate of wrinkling and loss of elasticity of the skin. Fasting from sugar is critical as well, and we'll discuss this more in a later chapter. But for now understand that sugar consumption plays a significant role in advancing the aging process and in the development or worsening of many degenerative diseases, such as diabetes, atherosclerosis, chronic renal failure, and Alzheimer's disease.[34] (Also see my book *The Juice Lady's Sugar Knockout* for help with kicking a sugar habit.)

Brightly colored fruits and vegetables contain antioxidants that fight advanced glycation end products (or AGEs) ("proteins or lipids that become glycated as a result of exposure to sugars"[35]) and harmful free radicals in the body. Also, fruits such as blueberries, noni, cranber-ries, and olives contain phytonutrients called iridoids, which have been shown to decrease the amount of AGEs in the body.

Fresh juices provide an abundance of phytonutrients that heal and restore cells. They also contain biophotons, which come from energy derived from the sun during photosynthesis. When living foods such as raw vegetables and fresh fruit are cooked, biophotons are destroyed. Biophotons help cells communicate more efficiently. And according to research from the University of Southern California, cycles of a four-day, low-calorie diet that mimicked fasting cut visceral belly fat, boosted neural regeneration, and improved learning and memory.[36] In short, fasting reverses brain aging and other aspects of the aging process. In another study subjects were put on twice-a-month, four-day, reduced-calorie fasts. Results showed the potential extension of life span, reduced incidence of cancer, stronger immune system, fewer inflammatory diseases, decreased bone-mineral-density loss, and improved cognitive abilities.[37] The diet called for a reduction in the individual's caloric intake, down to 34 to 54 percent of his or her usual consumption, with a customized combination of proteins, carbohydrates, fats, and micronutrients. The hormone IGF-I, a promoter of aging that also has been associated with cancer susceptibility, also decreased due to specifications in the diet.[38]

Do you need an antiaging intervention?

Recent aging research has looked for interventions that may help people avoid or slow the hands of Father Time. The quest for healthy aging and younger appearance, a state in which improved longevity is coupled with good health, is the most desirable outcome. Fasting, a healthy diet, and exercise regimens "have been shown to prolong life and/or sustain health late in life":

> Autophagy [a physiological process that deals with destruction of cells] up-regulation [an increase in the number of receptors on cells], improved stress resistance and mitochondrial efficiency are among the cellular functions needed to hold off features associated with accelerated aging, such as free radical generation, excess caloric intake, chronic hyperglycemia, and fat accumulation.[39]

Ann Wigmore, the founder of the Hippocrates Health Institute, offered a great example of someone who experienced the antiaging effects of fasting using raw foods that included sprouts and wheatgrass juice. She reported that "her energy improved, her gray hair turned dark again, and her sagging skin tightened as though she'd had a facelift."[40] She also cured an injured leg of gangrene and saved it from amputation.[41]

Fasting is one of the most natural, noninvasive, and healthy methods to roll back the years and improve your health at the same time. Fasting resides at the center of the natural approaches to antiaging. It is very safe, unlike surgery or Botox injections, and also unlike manipulation of the body, it affects our cells. Years ago I was told about an unpublished study of chicken cells that a professor had kept alive in her lab with a controlled type of nutrient-rich fast, during which she fed the cells superior nutrients and cleansed them frequently. While she was on vacation one time, her students failed to care for the cells properly. She returned to a shriveled-up experiment. Just when she was about to toss them, she had an idea to give them more nutrients and cleanse them even more frequently. They returned to their once soft, supple state. This is what fasting, especially juice fasting, can do for us.

A younger brain

A fast is a vacation for your digestive system and a boost for your brain. It's an opportunity for your body to clean out the wastes that have accumulated, including the brown slime called lipofuscin that can collect in the brain, causing dementia and Alzheimer's. Raw juices, as I mentioned earlier, provide scores of nutritional helpers in the form of antioxidants and phytonutrients that scavenge free radicals, thus preventing further damage to brain cells as well as helping the brain detox. They also offer other nutrients that repair and restore cells, soluble fibers that act as "internal brooms," and nutrient-rich water that flushes out accumulated wastes.

Fasting to improve brain function is not a new practice. As mentioned earlier, ancient Greek philosophers used fasting to improve their cognitive abilities. Do you think they were right? Think about the last big meal you ate. How did you feel afterward? Energetic? Mentally alert? Probably not. Most likely you felt wiped out and ready to take a nap. And you felt this way because your body had to gather blood from all around the body and assign it to the digestive system in order to handle the huge amount of food you just dropped on it. This leaves less blood going to the brain, which results in a sluggish, foggy, dreary brain in a state that is known as a "food coma."[42]

Many people who have joined my online juice-fast classes have reported that early on their foggy brain went away. "Research has indicated that fasting can significantly reduce the effects of aging on the brain.... Bouts of intermittent fasting... [are] one of the key strategies for maximizing brain function."[43] Indeed, not only have people in my groups reported that they got rid of brain fog, but they also experienced a sharper mind, better cognition, and better recall.

Scientists also have discovered that in animals such as mice reduced meal frequency appears to have "a protective effect on the brain and may also help with heart function and regulation of sugar content in the blood."[44]

At a symposium held at the Society for Neuroscience's annual meeting, researchers pointed to these brain-specific advantages of intermittent fasting:[45]

+ Increased synaptic plasticity (a biological marker of learning and memory)

+ Enhanced performance on memory tests in the elderly

+ Stimulated growth of new neurons

+ Promoted recovery after stroke or traumatic brain injury

+ Decreased risk of neurodegenerative diseases, such as Alzheimer's and Parkinson's, and potential improvement in the quality of life and cognitive function of those already diagnosed with these diseases

+ Preventative and therapeutic role in mood disorders such as anxiety and depression

The conclusion of this discussion at the symposium was this: as you periodically deprive your body of food in a well-managed way, you will see your brain and indeed your entire body come back stronger and more efficient. Your brain and body need to be challenged. If you think of it as you would weight training, then you'll understand that sometimes you have to break parts of your system down to see it built back up.

Begin to regenerate

Ultimately, when your brain is challenged by fasting, it adapts its stress-response pathways, just as it would if it were responding to regular exercise. Both fasting and exercise "increase the production of protein in the brain (neurotrophic factors), which in turn promotes the growth of neurons, the connection between neurons, and the strength of synapses."[46] Fasting also spurs new nerve cell and ketone production. This activity also may increase the number of mitochondria in neurons as a result of the brain's adapting to the stress (good stress) that fasting puts on the body. With a rising number of mitochondria in the neurons, the ability to learn and recall is improved.[47]

A study of chemotherapy patients who went for long periods without eating showed that their white-blood-cell counts dropped significantly.[48] This could mean that fasting helps the body terminate and shed ravaged immune cells. As the body restores itself, it manufactures brand-new cells from stem cells. Fasting promotes stem-cell-based regeneration.

Researcher Valter Longo said:

> When you starve [or fast for a few days], the system tries to save energy, and one of the things it can do to save energy is to recycle a lot of the immune cells that are not needed, especially those that may be damaged. What we started noticing in both our human work and animal work is that the white blood cell count goes down with prolonged fasting. Then when you re-feed, the blood cells come back.[49]

It also has been reported that fasting effectively decreases the risk of cardiovascular disease, cancer, diabetes, and inflammation, which is at the root of nearly all diseases and ailments.[50]

GRAB YOUR FAST AND LET'S GO!

The ancient discipline of fasting provides miraculous benefits to every part of your being, and because of this it is gaining popularity among researchers, health advocates, and people like you who want to live life to the fullest. So let's go deeper!

In the next chapter I'll explain the different types of fasts. You can choose the one that fits you best. Or, over time, you can sample each one. Why not? One-day fasts are a great way to get an idea about the different types of fasts available. Then you'll know which one provides you with the greatest benefits.

Get ready to fast for a new you!

Chapter 2

THE DIFFERENT FASTING DIETS

One way to begin to see how vastly indulgent we usually are is to fast. It is a long day that is not broken
by the usual three meals. One finds out what an astonishing amount of time is spent in the planning, pur-
chasing, preparing, eating, and cleaning up of meals.
—ELISABETH ELLIOT

ARE YOU EXCITED about finding the right fast for you? There are
a variety of wonderful fasts to choose from. This chapter is your
go-to chapter for discovering the different types of fasts available. We will cover the juice fast; a fasting combination of juices and
smoothies; the bone-broth fast; intermittent fasting; sugar fasting; and
the Daniel fast, which is also known as the Lenten fast or the vegan fast.
You may want to try them all for different reasons and different weeks
of fasting throughout the year. You could set aside a month of fasting
and choose a different type of fast each week. Or you could devote a few
days to juice fasting and then some days or even weeks to the other fasts.
Choose what will work for you. But no matter the choice, you will benefit greatly from trying these fasts.

THE JUICE FAST

A juice fast (or liquid diet, as some call it) is one in which you drink
only juices and liquids such as herbal tea, broth, and water. More than a
trend, juicing and juice fasting appear to be gaining in popularity. From
the red-carpet crowd to Main Street America, people from coast to

coast are discovering that juice fasting helps them reset their metabolism, revive—that is, "get their glow back"—lose weight, and restore health.

A juice fast is very safe. With all the juice-fast retreats and groups we have led, I have never had anyone experience a bad outcome. In fact, it's quite the opposite. I usually see very positive changes in just a few days. It's truly exciting for many people! We offer juice-and-raw-food retreats several times a year. We all juice-fast together for three days. By the end of the week it's amazing to hear about the many health improvements people have experienced. I've seen scores of people healed in five days. And as I mentioned earlier, most people lose between five and ten pounds during that time. I've also had people juice-fast who were very thin and needed to gain weight. Some people who were too thin actually put on a couple of pounds. The body will do what it needs to do when you give it a chance to heal.

Juice fasting is rewarding because it provides abundant nutrition while also supporting the digestive system, providing it with an opportunity to rest and heal. Many holistic practitioners have used juice fasting to help patients heal their bodies more speedily. When you aren't eating solid food all day long, your digestive system, and indeed your whole body, can work on other functions such as repair, restoration, and removal of dead cells. It's like having someone clean your house. Think about how much time that gives you for other things that need to get done.

It takes about six to eight hours for food to pass through your stomach and small intestine. According to the Mayo Clinic, researchers measured digestion in twenty-one healthy people, from start to finish—eating to elimination—and found it's about a fifty-three-hour journey.[1] But when you drink nutrient-rich juices, which are broken down into a highly digestible form that is absorbed easily, you're well fed without all that work. It's estimated that the nutrients from juicing are at work in your system within about thirty minutes. Voilà! You're nourished—with energy to spare for your personal reboot.

There is no restriction on the amount of juice you can drink on a juice fast. I do recommend, however, that most of the juice be vegetable juice and that you restrict fruit juice. You can overdo it on fruit juice and get too much sugar. Use fruit only to flavor and sweeten your drinks a bit.

Rather than feeling hungry during a juice fast, you should feel satisfied because your body is being well fed. If you have emotional hunger, see chapter 10 on emotional fasting. You may miss chewing and the desire for crunch. If you do feel ravenous, you might have an overgrowth of yeast or other parasites that are screaming for their favorite food.

You should feel lighter and more energized by the second or third day of a juice fast. But don't worry if that's not the case for you. You are probably detoxing. (See chapter 4 for more information on fasting and detoxing.)

How juice fasting benefits you

Here's why juice fasting is so powerful in changing how you feel and look:

Provides a gentle detox

Fresh, raw juice is rich in antioxidants that bind up toxins that would otherwise damage your cells. Without all those bad guys roaming around in your system, you'll have less damage to your cells. That means fewer wrinkles, a healthier brain, and a stronger immune system. It also means more repair from the inside out. You'll start looking younger and more vibrant. You'll improve the health of your stomach and intestinal tract. Are you hooked on antacids? Trouble with digestion? Juice fasting and bone-broth fasting can give your stomach a break, as it won't have to work so hard to extract nutrients. That's because the initial work of breaking down the food so your body can utilize the nutrients is done by the juicer. If you have low stomach acid—which can cause acid reflux—you'll get relief. You won't need as much strong acid to break down the juices. And after the juice cleanse, you could try adding 2 teaspoons of raw apple-cider vinegar to 6 ounces of water and drinking it fifteen minutes before you eat. That may solve your acid-reflux problem.

Repairs your gut

That's right! Gut repair is possible. The standard American diet is a gut buster for sure, and not in the best sense of that phrase. Here's how the gut gets damaged. The American diet is replete with damaged fats, sugars, and other refined carbs such as white-flour products that turn to glue-like substances in the gut, along with gooey cheese and foods saturated in additives and pesticides. Down those with soda or a sugary drink, and dump on that conglomeration some antacids and other over-the-counter drugs, and you have an irritating, congesting, gut-damaging mess. Then twist it all up with a heaping dose of stress, and you have more than enough to give you constant indigestion and do damage to the tiny microvilli in your intestinal tract that are responsible for nutrient absorption. This can lead to leaky-gut syndrome, which allows larger particles of food to escape and float into your system. Leaky gut is responsible for a number of health issues, including food allergies.

Rejuvenates your liver

Your liver is the king of your detoxification organs. It's the hardest-working organ you have. Everything has to pass through your liver. It's the prep plant for the rest of the body. Problems arise when there are too many toxins for the liver to deal with. It can get congested and even develop stones, just like the gallbladder.

Fatty liver disease is the up-and-coming condition for younger and younger people. That's because we eat far too much sugar—about 20 teaspoons a day for the average person. Fasting takes you into a sugar-free zone in which you can begin to heal the liver and get rid of the fatty liver.

Now is the time to cleanse this key organ. It's key to your health, to youthfulness, and to efficient weight loss.

Accelerates weight loss

As I've already mentioned, you can lose five to ten pounds in a week when you juice-fast. I say this because I can back it up with stories from all the people who have attended our juice-fast retreats through the years and people who have signed up for my online juice-fast and detox programs. You will lose some water weight, but what's wrong with that? You also will lose fat. The three- to five-day juice cleanse is a fantastic way to jump-start your detox. It helps you control cravings. I call it the ultimate palate cleanse. Because your juice-fast days are lower in calories (usually around 600–800 or less when you don't use a lot of fruit), you will lose weight. But you aren't starving your body because you're also receiving plenty of healing, energizing nutrients.

Flattens your belly

Watch your stomach shrink with a juice fast. You'll get rid of belly bloat and fat in short order. That muffin top will melt away day by day.

Kicks up your energy

The first day or two of a juice fast you may not have more energy; you may be more tired as toxins are released. But just wait! Energy is on its way—and this energy is better than anything you get from caffeine, energy drinks, or sugar. This is true, sustaining energy.

Improves mental clarity

Juice fasting/cleansing is the ultimate foggy-brain buster. You might feel a little spacey at the start of a juice fast, but then the fog will clear, and those 100-billion-plus little neurons in your brain will spark up. One reason for the better clarity is that you're restricting calories. A study published in the journal *Neurobiology of Aging* found "there is significant evidence linking caloric restriction in adult mice with the growth of new brain cells.... Specifically it is linked to increased production of BDNF [brain-derived neurotrophic factor]. Basically restricting your calories and not overeating produces somewhat of a stress response in the body. Following this stress response is the production of new neurons."[2]

Heals your body at the cellular level

When you flood your system with raw juices, you provide an abundance of biophotons, which are light rays of energy that plants absorb from the sun. They help your cells communicate better. And when you start cleansing the interstitial fluids that bathe the cells, your little cells start taking in nutrients and expelling waste more efficiently. Biophotons also feed your mitochondria, the energy units of your cells. All this spells—you guessed it—cellular healing.

Provides maximum nutrient replenishment

As you drink your nutrient-charged fresh raw juices, you are consuming a cornucopia of nutrients: antioxidants, vitamins, minerals, enzymes, phytonutrients, and biophotons. Your body uses all these raw materials for detoxification, which means now your body can support all the phases of detoxification far more efficiently. Plus, you won't be pouring in more toxins. On a normal day many people consume congestive and/or toxic substances all day long. The body can barely keep up with what's coming down the pipes, let alone clear out stored-up toxic material. It's kind of like a heavy snowstorm. You may shovel all day long just to keep your deck from collapsing. Finally you're worn out and collapse on the couch. (That happened to us one March day in Colorado with a heavy early spring blizzard!)

During your juice-fast days your body can focus on removing the cumulative toxins stored in organs, cells, and tissue spaces—and for most of us, there's a lot of unwanted material stored up:

> In a study spearheaded by the Environmental Working Group (EWG) in collaboration with Commonweal, researchers at two major laboratories found an average of 200 industrial chemicals and pollutants in umbilical cord blood from 10 babies born in August and September of 2004 in U.S. hospitals. Tests revealed a total of 287 chemicals in the group. The umbilical cord blood of these 10 children, collected by Red Cross after the cord was cut, harbored pesticides, consumer product ingredients, and wastes from burning coal, gasoline, and garbage.[3]

If newborn babies have 200-plus chemicals at birth, what about the rest of us? It is obvious that we all need plenty of detoxifying, antioxidant-rich juices and foods. That's why juice fasting, with all its easily absorbed nutrients, is so powerful.

Purges mucus

Do you have mucus hanging out in your inner parts? The juice fast, like no other form of fasting, helps your body get rid of excess mucus that can build up over time. Various mucous membranes line body cavities and canals in the body, such as the respiratory, digestive, and urogenital tracts. They are found in the mouth, nose, trachea, eyelids, lungs, stomach, intestines, and bladder. Mucus provides protection and lubrication, and it offers a barrier from outside invaders.

When we're in a state of good health, this mucus has a thin consistency. But over time, with a buildup of toxins, it can change. We may experience a buildup of thicker mucus, which can clog our systems, muck up our throats, harbor chemicals and pathogens, and trap dead cells that would otherwise be removed. When we juice fast, we eliminate refined-flour products, fried foods, sugar, dairy, soda, caffeine, alcohol, fast food, and junk food—typical mucus-forming foods and substances. As we ditch the irritating foods and substances, the body stops producing excess mucus, and what's then produced is more of a normal consistency. The body can work on sweeping out the old, thick mucus, dead cells, pathogens, and other foreign matter.

Alkalizes

This is another juicy bonus. Fresh juices are very alkaline and help balance the pH in your body. You must maintain a delicate, precise pH balance in the blood, which is slightly alkaline. A healthy pH balance should be between 7.35 and 7.45. To maintain this delicate range, the body will draw minerals from bones, teeth, and muscles to use as buffers against the acids if there aren't enough minerals present in your diet.

The acidity or alkalinity of foods can be classified by how we process them. Our bodies transform nearly all foods into acid or alkaline bases. Though we need a balance of different foods for good health, most people eat far more acid-producing foods than alkaline-forming foods. Consuming excess acid-producing substances causes a condition called acidosis.

Adding high-alkaline foods and vegetable juices to your diet brings your pH into better balance. You will notice that you gain energy when your body is more alkaline balanced. Fresh juices are packed with minerals and other nutrients that help you achieve this goal.

Enjoying a Clearer Mind

"After the first few days of juice fasting, I feel much clearer minded. Prayer time was much clearer as well." —Jena

Think you don't have time?

As Dr. Cynthia Foster says, "Neither do I, but I still do it."[4] In an ideal situation we'd drink the juice we make right after we juice it. However, for those on a crunched schedule, you can make it the night before and store it in the refrigerator, and then take it with you in a cooler the next day. You also can make a big batch on the weekend and freeze the juice in individual jars—just be sure to leave some room at the top for it to expand when it freezes, or the jar will break.

Juice bars are becoming more common, so you can pick up healthy juices on the go. You can also, in a pinch, drink a low-sodium V8.

Fresh juice vs. store-bought juice

Speaking of low-sodium V8, people often ask me why they should go to the trouble of making their own juice. Why not just buy it? After all, stores are now stocked with a growing array of bottled juices made from organic ingredients. You can even find them with kale, beets, and ginger.

The primary reason you want to make your own juice is that you can't get the same nutritional benefits from store-bought juice. Many of the popular brands of juice have been pasteurized, which is required by law, so the juice is missing most of the original vitamins, enzymes, and biophotons, as they're killed off when the juice is heated.

But high-pressure processing (HPP) is an option. HPP involves a "high level of cool pressure [that] is applied evenly to destroy any pathogens and ensure the juice is safe to drink."[5] The HPP process preserves vitamins, minerals, phytonutrients, and enzymes. You'll find these juices in stores such as Whole Foods and from brands such as Suja Elements.

How about more variety? This is another good reason to make your own juice. The store-bought brews limit you to the best sellers. If you make your own juices and smoothies, you can pick a variety of dark greens that are nutrient dense and produce that is local, fresh, and organic. You can make unusual drinks with herbs such as basil or mint, use flowers such as lavender and fennel, enjoy spices such as fresh turmeric and ginger, and even add horseradish (a root veggie used as spice). Once your taste buds hit your homemade fresh elixir, you may never want store-bought juice again.

Take a quick look at chapter 7 for juice-fast menus and recipes. There you'll find recipes using yummy ingredients more varied and numerous than you will ever find at your corner store. And once you get accustomed to making fresh juice, you can branch out and start creating your own favorite combinations. The vitamins, minerals, enzymes, phytochemicals, and biophotons extracted from nature's best will energize your body and give you a feeling of well-being almost instantly. And talk about getting rid of sluggishness! That will exit with the toxins. Get ready to raise your beautiful glass with a toast to your health.

Detoxing at Age Sixty-Eight

"I am writing to let you know that I just finished a twenty-one-day juice fast using organic carrots, kale, fine herbs, a bit of pineapple, and Essiac tea. The Lord led me to start this fast before discovering that my husband had purchased your books after hearing you on Sid Roth's program. After fourteen days on the fast I ordered your book on juice fasting, which was very helpful.

"A few weeks before starting the fast I had been tested by a naturopathic doctor. I made an appointment with her to be retested the last day of my twenty-one-day fast. She had never seen so much improvement with a client in just a month! I am encouraged and determined to pursue my effort to detox at sixty-eight years old! I thank God for your insights, depth of research on the subject, and your persistence in helping people to better understand and respect God's design of our bodies as well as keeping the temple of the Holy Spirit cleaned—physically, emotionally, and spiritually." —Brenda

Ready, set…go!

Preparation is the key to fasting success. Get ready for your juice fast ahead of time. Check the recipes in chapter 7 that you want to try. Make your shopping list, and get all your produce before your start date. Buy enough supplies to last for the duration of your fast if you can, unless you have a prolonged fast. If you are missing items, your kickoff may be delayed, and you may get discouraged and lose your enthusiasm. You might even ditch the whole thing. Also assemble your equipment. Make sure your juicer is in working order.

Set your mind to prepare in advance. I've found this is a very important step. If I tell myself I can do it, I always do much better than if I waffle about doing it. Also, without all the "emotional food stuffers"— snacks and treats—you may notice how often you want to stress-eat or eat out of boredom, loneliness, frustration, irritation, or a myriad of other emotions. If you frequently desire to do this, you may want to go on an emotional fast and purge your toxic emotions, which you can learn how to do in chapter 10.

If this is the first time you are juice fasting and you are overcome with hunger by the end of the day, you could eat a raw salad. Use only lemon juice and olive oil for a dressing. If you feel weak and shaky and have to work, you could make a green smoothie with avocado. Then continue with your juice fast the next day. If you have gnawing hunger, you may have parasites, in which case you would want to consider a parasite cleanse. (See the Resources appendix.)

Now, go for it! Make this a renewing, rejuvenating juice fast.

Supplies You'll Need

- **Juicer.** Plug it in and go!
- **Produce.** Choose organic, as you don't want to pour a lot of toxic pesticides into your body when you're trying to purge them out.
- **Glass jars.** Use these if you plan to freeze juice ahead of time.
- **Purified water.** Don't forget to drink plenty of water when you're juice fasting. See chapter 3 about the importance of drinking water, especially when you fast.

THE LEMONADE FAST (AKA MASTER CLEANSE)

The lemonade fast—or master cleanse, as many people call it—is a lemon-juice fast. Its popularity began in 1940, with millions of people all over the world claiming success with it.

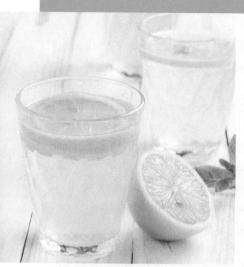

Here's the recipe:

2 Tbsp. fresh-squeezed lemon juice
2 Tbsp. pure organic maple syrup (or
a few drops of liquid stevia)
Pinch of cayenne pepper
2 cups purified water
Dark, leafy greens (optional)

For the lemonade fast you should drink between six and twelve glasses of this lemonade a day. Whenever you feel hungry, grab a glass of it.

Here's my recommendation for this recipe and fast: Maple syrup is high in sugar, so I'd recommend a few drops of liquid stevia (an herbal sweetener) instead because it's lower on the glycemic index. You need only a few drops because it is very sweet. My favorite brand and flavor is SweetLeaf Vanilla Crème.

You also may want to make green lemonade if you're going to try the lemonade fast. You could juice lemons with some dark, leafy greens such as chard or kale. This is a much healthier choice and will accomplish your cleansing goal with better nutrition.

On this program it is recommended that you take a laxative before bed. I like the Digestive Stimulator by Blessed Herbs or ColonMax by Advanced Naturals. (See the Resources appendix.) Here's why you want to keep your bowels moving: because fresh lemon juice is known to help oxygenate the body, support enzyme functions, and stimulate liver enzymes, the liver will start dumping toxins, such as uric acid. This fast is known for stirring up a great deal of waste. The toxins will come pouring out of fat cells, the liver, and tissue spaces. It will also work on clearing congested bile ducts. It can help in removing calcium deposits. It helps clear deposits from the kidneys and pancreas. When the body begins to dump all this toxic waste, you want your colon clear and ready to remove the waste as efficiently as possible. This will help to prevent uncomfortable detox symptoms. This is why a saltwater flush is recommended on the master cleanse—to move the waste out fast. Though this part of the cleanse is optional, it is highly recommended.

Saltwater Flush

2 tsp. sea salt, pink Himalayan salt, or grey salt
4 cups purified water

Mix the salt with the water. Drink the entire solution in five minutes. Lie on your right side for thirty minutes to allow the water to pass through. Hold until your body is ready to eliminate.

It might be good to do this saltwater flush in the evening, when you have time at home. You have to have one to seven bowel movements. If you don't like the taste of saltwater—and really, who does?—chug it on down quickly. You can chase it with plain water.

JUICE-AND-SMOOTHIE FAST

Whereas fresh juice comes from running produce through a juicer, with the fiber being ejected into a pulp catcher, a smoothie is a blend of foods that are made into a thick shake using the whole ingredients—although with some produce, such as oranges and avocados, you need to remove the skin, and with other produce, such as avocados and peaches, you need to remove the seed before making a smoothie.

Smoothies contain *all* the fiber. Also, they are more filling than juices. Some people have a challenge drinking only juice, especially on workdays; therefore supplementing with smoothies and raw soups makes it possible to do an all-liquid fast and still work. The juice fast is the one that seems to bring about the most change for myself and others, but many people seem to need something extra in their diet, especially when they work.

Green smoothies made from nutrient-rich, dark-green vegetables are the best for those who are watching both their weight and the glycemic load in their daily diets. They are great when you want to include ingredients such as plant milk (coconut, almond, or hemp, for example), protein powder, nuts, seeds, or organic tofu.

You can combine juice, smoothies, broth, and raw soups to make a liquid fast that has more sustaining properties. For the menu plan and recipes, see chapter 7.

THE DANIEL FAST (LENTEN FAST, VEGAN FAST)

A spiritual fast based on the Bible's Book of Daniel, the Daniel fast refers to either a ten-day or a twenty-one-day period of abstaining from all animal foods and wine. It includes eating vegan foods only and is based on biblical accounts of foods that encourage health. This fast is also sometimes called the "Lenten fast" or the "vegan fast."

With a popular fast named after him, aren't you just a bit curious about who Daniel was? He was among the brightest and best of young Israeli men chosen by King Nebuchadnezzar to serve in his Babylonian palace. King Nebuchadnezzar seized Judah's capital city of Jerusalem, captured King Jehoiakim, and destroyed the Israelites' temple of worship. He then took the brightest and best of the young men from wealthy, influential Israeli families—those who were strong, handsome, and intelligent and who demonstrated good leadership abilities—and entered them into a three-year training program in preparation to serve him.

Daniel and his friends were among the young men chosen for this honor, and they were to be given the king's gourmet food and wine that came from his own table. Most historians agree the food included unclean animals that had been sacrificed to idols. But Daniel asked the chief official in charge of them if he and his friends could have just pulse and water—a diet that was according to Jewish custom. In biblical accounts *pulse* means herbs and vegetables. According to *Smith's Bible Dictionary*, it included seeds and usually legumes such as dried peas, beans, and the seeds that grow in pods, and would include lentils and grains such as barley, wheat, and millet.[6]

Daniel 1:12–13 (KJV) gives the account:

Prove thy servants, I beseech thee, ten days; and let them give us pulse to eat, and water to drink. Then let our countenances be looked upon before thee, and the countenance of the children that eat of the portion of the king's meat: and as thou seest, deal with thy servants.

At first Daniel simply had asked that he not be forced to defile himself with the king's food, but the official was not for the idea, not wanting Daniel and his friends to look frail or unhealthy and catch the wrath of the king. So they made a deal with the guard: "Give us our vegan diet and water for ten days, and then compare how we look with the way the other young men appear. Judge our diet according to what you see." To this the guard acquiesced.

After ten days the men were brought before the king. Their health and appearance were better than the health and appearance of all the young men who consumed the finest from the king's table. Three years later, and still eating the same diet, Daniel was ten times better than all the king's magicians and astrologers (Dan. 1:18–20).

Daniel outlived King Nebuchadnezzar and became an adviser to his descendant Belshazzar. And in his later years Daniel still fasted, once for twenty-one days in mourning for the Jewish people, based on a vision he received from God. Daniel 10:2–3 says, "At that time I, Daniel, mourned for three weeks. I ate no choice food; no meat or wine touched my lips; and I used no lotions at all until the three weeks were over" (NIV).

As you can see, fasting was a key to Daniel's success and survival in a foreign and hostile land. Daniel lived a fasted life but also had periods he devoted to fasting and prayer. Those periods were life-changing. His example is one reason the Daniel fast is so popular today.

Here's what you can drink and eat on a Daniel Fast

This is a general guideline for what you can choose to drink and eat on your Daniel fast. Chapter 8 gives you a menu plan and plenty of recipes for breakfast, lunch, and dinner.

Beverages

On the Daniel fast you can drink purified water, spring water, distilled water, or sparkling water. You can have herbal tea or green tea. You can enjoy coconut water, coconut kefir, coconut milk, almond milk, hemp milk, and rice milk (no soy milk; it is not a healthy choice). Vegetable juices or veggie juices flavored with a little fruit are also acceptable.

Fruit (eat moderately—one to two servings per day)

According to the United States Department of Agriculture (USDA) a serving of fruit is "1 cup of fruit or 100% fruit juice, or 1/2 cup of dried fruit."[7]

The fruit can be fresh, frozen, dried, dehydrated, or juiced. (Eat no canned fruit.) I recommend you choose mostly low-sugar fruits such as berries (blackberries, blueberries, boysenberries, raspberries, strawberries, cranberries), green apples, lemons, limes, tomatoes, avocados, and pears. But all fruits are part of this fast. Make sure, however, that you juice mostly vegetables rather than fruit. As I've already mentioned, straight fruit juice is very high in sugar. It is better to eat the fruit whole and use just a little bit of low-sugar fruit to flavor and sweeten your juice recipes. Personally I use lemon and lime for my juices, but no other fruit. If you choose dried fruits, make sure there are no added sulfites, oils, or sugar.

Vegetables (eat at least five servings of vegetables a day)

According to the USDA a serving of vegetables is "1 cup of raw or cooked vegetables or vegetable juice, or 2 cups of raw leafy greens."[8]

Vegetables can be fresh, frozen, dried, dehydrated, or juiced. (Use no canned veggies.) Veggie burgers are also a good choice, but avoid all veggie burgers that contain soy.

Whole grains (eat moderately—two to three servings per day)

According to the USDA a serving of grains includes "1 slice of bread, 1 cup of ready-to-eat cereal, or 1/2 cup of cooked rice, cooked pasta, or cooked cereal."[9]

No leavened bread—that is, bread made with yeast—is allowed. If you are not gluten sensitive, choose only organic whole wheat to avoid the unhealthy pesticides sprayed on wheat just before harvesting. I'm not a fan of wheat, since I've found many people to be sensitive to it and not aware that it is causing problems for them. I recommend ancient grains. You can choose brown, red, green, or black rice (try green rice; it's really good), as well as millet, buckwheat, teff, Kamut, quinoa, oats, barley, and rye. I suggest quinoa or brown-rice pasta, brown-rice crackers, and organic popcorn.

Nuts and seeds

If you don't want to put on weight, limit seeds and nuts to no more than two dozen nuts, 2 tablespoons of seeds, or 1 tablespoon of nut or seed butters per day. Nuts and seeds can be fattening for some people because they contain a lot of fat and some carbs.

Choose sprouted, raw, or dry-roasted nuts or seeds. (Sprouted nuts are the healthiest.) Pumpkin and watermelon seeds help to kill parasites; they are excellent choices. Peanuts are not actually nuts but rather a legume. They are prone to molds and not as healthy a choice. Nut and seed butters are also a good choice, but avoid brands with added sugar. My favorite is the nut butter I grind fresh at the health-food store. Many health-food stores have that option.

Legumes—beans, lentils, split peas

According to the USDA a 1-ounce serving is 1/4 cup of cooked beans (such as black, kidney, pinto, or white beans), 1/4 cup of cooked peas (such as chickpeas, cowpeas, lentils, or split peas), and 1/4 cup of baked beans and refried beans.[10]

Choose legumes that are dried and cooked in water or canned as long as there are no additives. Strive for 1 to 2 cups of legumes a day on this fast; they provide protein.

Oil

When it comes to oils, you can have extra-virgin olive oil, organic virgin coconut oil, grapeseed oil, almond oil, avocado oil, macadamia nut oil, and sesame oil. Avoid all other oils, including canola, safflower, sunflower, corn, and soy.

(Please note: The Orthodox Lenten fast does not include oil.)

Condiments

You may have raw apple-cider vinegar, sea salt, fresh herbs, and spices.

Foods to avoid on the Daniel Fast

While there's plenty you can eat on the Daniel fast, there's also plenty you can't eat. Let's consider the options that are—quite literally—off the table when you're on this fast.

Meat and other animal products

Avoid all meat and other animal products on the Daniel fast, including but not limited to beef, lamb, pork, poultry, fish, and eggs.

Dairy

Avoid all dairy products, including but not limited to milk, cheese, cream, buttermilk, yogurt, and butter.

Sweeteners

Avoid all sugar, including but not limited to maple syrup, raw sugar, honey, syrups, molasses, brown-rice syrup, and cane juice. You may use stevia, which is an herb. For a complete list of all types of sugar and what's healthy and what's not, see chapter 8, "The Sugar Shopping Guide," in my book *The Juice Lady's Sugar Knockout*.

Leavened bread

This includes all baked goods and even Ezekiel bread, which contains yeast.

Refined and processed foods

Avoid all refined and processed foods that contain artificial flavors, colors, dyes, preservatives, and other chemicals. Avoid all white flour and white rice. Choose only whole foods.

Fried foods

This includes tortilla chips, potato chips, corn chips, French fries, tempura, and all types of deep-fried foods.

Stimulating beverages

Avoid all coffee, black tea, sodas, energy drinks, and alcohol, including beer, wine, and hard liquor.

Bone-Broth Fast

Bone broth is the nation's hottest brew these days. Some people are doing bone-broth fasts, while others are adding bone broth to other types of fasts, such as the juice fast. The bone-broth diet isn't something new; it's just rediscovered. It's been around for as long as people have boiled bones for soup stock. It's known to reverse signs of aging, promote weight loss, increase energy, decrease joint pain, and renew vitality—in just twenty-one days. It can help heal your gut because it reduces inflammation. It's amazingly nutritious for your joints and bones.

If you go on the bone-broth diet, know that it is basically a modified Paleo Diet that involves avoiding sugar, all grains, and most high-carbohydrate foods while fasting two days a week on bone broth. You can go on this two-day-a-week fast program indefinitely. People have used this diet to help reduce inflammation, improve gut health, and shed pounds. I have included a similar diet with a twenty-eight-day menu plan, to which you could add bone broth, in *The Juice Lady's Anti-Inflammation Diet*. Dr. Kellyann Petrucci has taken this diet mainstream. She adds lots and lots of bone broth to the basic Paleo Diet.

For the fast days of this diet you will consume only bone broth. For the healthiest broth be sure to make (or purchase ready-made) broth from the bones of grass-fed cows or pastured chickens and from collagen-rich bones such as the neck, feet, and femur. The bone-broth fast is excellent for resetting your metabolism, decreasing inflammation, improving blood-glucose levels, and putting your body into a state of ketosis, meaning your body is burning fat for energy rather than glucose.

Slow cooking draws out collagen, amino acids (glycine, glucosamine, arginine, proline, and glutamine), and minerals such as calcium and magnesium. Bone broth is considered a superfood. It's known for improving skin,

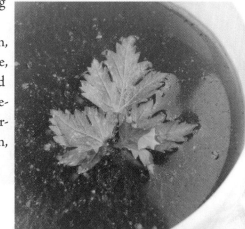

hair, and nails; giving your digestion a boost; and healing joints that ache.

Why is this broth so healthy for the joints? Dr. Josh Axe says, "One of the most valuable components of bone broth is gelatin, which acts like a soft cushion between bones that helps them 'glide' without friction. Gelatin also provides us with building blocks that are needed to form and maintain strong bones, helping take pressure off of aging joints and supporting healthy bone mineral density."[11] Also he reports, "Research done by the Department of Nutrition and Sports Nutrition for Athletics at Penn State University found that when athletes supplemented with collagen over the course of 24 weeks, the majority showed significant improvements in joint comfort and a decrease in factors that negatively impacted athletic performance."[12]

You can combine bone-broth fasting with juice fasting. The two are more powerful combined but can be combined only with a bone-broth protein powder if you are mixing the two together. Jordan Rubin, who has studied the health benefits of bone broth, says, "Bone Broth contains powerful nutrients and beneficial compounds to enhance digestion and detoxification. Since Bone Broth can't be added in a liquid form to veggie juice as it will greatly dilute the juice, there has not been a way to combine these amazing superfoods until now. By adding concentrated Bone Broth Protein to veggie or fruit juice, you can infuse the juice with protein and collagen, which can slow the absorption of the sugars contained in the juice and enhance the juice with nutrients the body craves."[13]

For the recipe for bone broth, see chapter 8.

INTERMITTENT FASTING

The two-day fast has become quite popular in recent years. Sporadic fasting is part of the history of mankind but probably not by choice in years past. Best-selling books have promoted this type of fast, as have actors, including Hugh Jackman and Benedict Cumberbatch. Talk-show host Jimmy Kimmel says he has followed this type of fasting diet for two years and that it has led to significant weight loss.[14]

Intermittent fasting is based on an intake of about 600 calories for men and 500 calories for women on each of the two days of intermittent fasting. That's equivalent to about three 10-ounce glasses of vegetable juice per day or two very-low-calorie meals with a mini snack.

You may have animal protein with this type of fast. In fact, research has found that people stay fuller longer if they have some protein. Usually the calories on this fast are packed into an eight-hour period of time, leaving sixteen hours for fasting. Based on scientific research, this type of fast has been found to work for many things, including weight loss, rebooting the brain, regenerating new nerve cells in the hippocampus, mood enhancement, gene repair, rest for the pancreas leading to improved insulin sensitivity, and stem-cell regeneration in general.[15] In another study the intermittent fast group experienced "decreases in tension, anger, confusion, and total mood disturbance and improvements in vigor."[16] And the intermittent-fasting groups typically lost more fat than the restricted-calorie-intake groups did.

This type of eating is effective because it puts your body through the opposite of what's normal. On a normal food-intake day the entire time you are eating and drinking, "your body is stuck in fat-storing mode....Only after a few hours of fasting is your body able to turn off the 'fat-storing' and turn on the 'fat-burning mechanisms.'"[17] The intermittent fast puts you in the fat-burning mode.

The two fast days can be done back to back or on different days of the week. You could also try what's called alternate-day fasting (ADF), which involves fasting every other day for two days and has also been found to be successful:

> Krista Varady, an associate professor of nutrition at the University of Illinois at Chicago, has studied the effects of alternate-day fasting on hundreds of obese adults. In trials lasting eight to 10 weeks, she has found that people lose on average about 13 pounds and experience marked reductions in LDL cholesterol, blood pressure, triglycerides and insulin, the fat-storage hormone.[18]

There is also time-restricted eating, which means packing all your meals in a six- to eight-hour window, leaving the remaining sixteen to eighteen hours in a day for fasting. On the benefits of this, "studies of time-restricted feeding practices in both animals and humans have suggested that the practice may lower cancer risk and help people maintain their weight."[19]

THE SUGAR FAST—A UNIVERSAL OPTION

If, for whatever reason, you can't do any of the other fasts reviewed in this chapter, you can fast from sugar and the foods that turn to sugar easily. None of us need sweet treats, sugary lattes, or refined-flour products. So this is a fast, or a portion of the fast, that every man, woman, and child can do.

Many people are addicted to sugar. We use sugar as a comfort food, a mood enhancer, a quick-jolt energizer, and a pick-me-up when we're bored. Now is the time to get rid of all sugar in its many forms—from honey to the white stuff. The only permissible sweetener is stevia, an herbal sweetener, or coconut sugar. No artificial sweeteners are allowed, either. In addition, avoid all refined carbohydrates, which includes all white-flour products. That means no buns, rolls, breads, crackers, pizza crust, pasta made with wheat flour, or flour tortillas. You also will be avoiding starch, such as white potatoes, but you may have sweet potatoes, purple potatoes, and yams. You also will avoid all alcohol.

When I was a child, I was very addicted to sugar. I'd eat sweets such as ice cream and cake with gooey frosting until they were gone. Do you remember the frosting made with Crisco and powdered sugar? I used to eat that stuff by the spoonful right out of the mixing bowl. Yikes! I was emotionally addicted as well as physically hooked. It is said that some sugar addictions are an attempt to bring sweetness into one's life. I think that was true for me, or at least the reason my sugar addiction started. My mother died when I was six years old. Her death was a tremendous loss because she was a wonderful mother. Her nickname was Honey—an appropriate name for one of the sweetest people I've ever known. Sadly nothing sweet could bring her back, and it was a poor comfort food in the end.

In order to completely let go of that addiction, I had to fast completely from sweets. I had to do this to get well. And I continue the sugar fast to this day to *stay* well. I live a fasted lifestyle. It's my path of wholeness.

For more information on how to give sugar the boot and detox from sweets, see my book *The Juice Lady's Sugar Knockout*. You also may want to join my sugar-detox group. (See www.juiceladycherie.com/Juice/30-day-detox for more information.)

LENGTHS OF FASTS

How long do you want to fast? You have many choices for the number of days you will alter your diet and the type of fast you can choose. You may want to try a variety of fasts during the year. Whatever you choose, I know you will benefit a great deal.

The one-day fast

If you have never fasted before, the one-day fast is the place you may want to start, especially if you are trying a water fast or juice fast. You can try the easy approach: start fasting after lunch on Friday, and end your fast twenty-four hours later with dinner on Saturday.

The two-day fast

As we discussed, the two-day fast is most often associated with the intermittent fast. There are many people who make the two-day fast part of their lifestyle. Again, you can fast two consecutive days or two days apart on this type of fast. It is based on 500 calories for women and 600 calories for men on the two days of fasting. (See the section on intermittent fasting for more information.) Of course, you can also do a two-day fast during which you don't take into account the exact number of calories you consume. Or you can do a two-day juice fast or juice-and-smoothie fast. You may also follow the vegan diet.

The three-day fast

I've been doing three-day juice fasts for more than two decades. We offer three-day veggie-juice fasts at our juice-and-raw-foods retreats. The retreats actually offer a five-day fast that's bookended with gourmet raw foods. Three days of juice fasting is not difficult for most people, especially when they are in a group. I also offer three- to five-day juice-fast groups that are part of the first week kickoff of my thirty-day detox.

The five-day fast

As I've already mentioned, I kicked off my health journey with a five-day juice fast. If I had not done that fast, I might not be here today helping you. Over and over again I've seen miracles happen with five-day fasts. I offer a five-day juice-fast program once a month that includes Facebook coaching and a conference call for questions and answers. (See the Resources appendix for more information.)

The seven-day fast

Make it a full week of fasting for a week of rejuvenation! With this approach you could combine juice fasting with smoothies and raw or cooked vegan meals for part of the week. Consider it a week's vacation for your body and soul.

The twenty-one-day fast

The twenty-one-day fast is the fast Daniel is known for. Today it's called the Daniel fast or vegan fast. You can make part or all of this fast juice fasting, but most people choose to follow primarily a vegan diet. (See chapter 8 for more on the Daniel fast.) The bone-broth diet or fast can be done for twenty-one days as well.

The thirty-day fast

Throughout the year I offer a thirty-day detox program that is a combination of a three- to five-day juice fast and then a vegan diet fast for the rest of the time. Many people have experienced incredible changes in their bodies during this thirty-day program. We go through the organs of elimination, starting with the three- to five-day juice fast and colon cleanse. In week two we focus on the liver-gallbladder cleanse with a parasite cleanse. Week three includes the kidney-bladder cleanse and lung detox. In week four we work on the lymphatic system and skin and blood. (For more information, see the Resources appendix.)

The Forty-day Fast

The forty-day fast is what Jesus embarked on as He went into the desert. Many church groups all over the United States and other parts of the world do a corporate forty-day Daniel fast in January, as the first part of the year is a great time to cleanse the body from all the effects of holiday excess. This type of fast is also known as the Lenten Fast in many liturgical churches and represents the forty days Jesus fasted after He was baptized.

ONE LAST NOTE

Many times I've heard people say they didn't feel well while fasting. Some fasting coaches indicate you must be doing something wrong if you aren't feeling great. That couldn't be further from the truth! You are probably detoxing when you feel this way. Giving up a lot of junk food and foods that are harder to digest, such as meat and dairy, allows your body to begin the wonderful work of cleansing.

This is a great opportunity to get rid of the stuff that could make you really sick down the road, susceptible to serious disease. So don't be alarmed if you get a few unwanted symptoms. Better a headache, a rash, or a bit of nausea now than cancer or diabetes or something equally alarming later on. I've devoted chapters 4 and 5 to this subject.

But first we'll look at water—both the water fast and the importance of drinking water when you fast.

Chapter 3

WATER AND FASTING

Water is the driving force of all nature.
—LEONARDO DA VINCI

F YOU'RE WONDERING what water fasting is all about, it is a dramatic fast that consists of your consuming only water. Many adherents of natural hygiene believe it is the only true method of fasting.

Water fasting is something I recommend for short fasts of one to three days. Beyond that, it can be physically challenging. Most people cannot remain on this type of fast for extended periods of time without adverse physical effects. The maximum amount of time I would recommend is one to two weeks, but that could be pushing it for some people, depending on their level of toxicity or physical strength.

I have never completed a water fast by choice. But I've done quite a few water fasts when, due to food poisoning or some other illness, I was unable to eat anything for several days. In the aftermath of that kind of devastation in my body I wanted only water. And even then I usually felt like eating again after one to three days. In any other circumstance I would not choose water fasting, and I'll tell you a couple of reasons why.

Years ago I interned under a nutritional, holistic, and medical doctor. He was working with a patient who was terribly out of balance and ill because of a water fast. He told me it would take about two years to get her back to health.

Although water fasting has been effective for some people when done for very short periods of time, Dr. Cynthia Foster, an expert in natural and holistic therapies, says that a water-only fast may be too harsh for most people's bodies to handle. "Some people," she says, "have reported that they never gained back their energy after doing a water fast."[1]

Water fasting can cause detoxification to occur too quickly, and during a water fast nutrients are not being replaced to help build up the systems that are being flushed. Antioxidants are not provided either to bind to toxins so they don't damage cells. Though this rapid breakdown of toxins can be initially beneficial, if the fast is sustained too long, the body will begin to catalyze muscle tissue once energy reserves from fat are consumed. This is when damage can take place.

In her article Dr. Foster told the story of a patient who refused to have anything to do with fasting. This patient was the sister of a previously healthy twenty-something man whose heart stopped suddenly during an extended water fast. The brother had no personal or generational history of heart problems. His death came as a complete shock to the family.[2] This is one example of why I caution people against strict water fasting for extended periods of time. Our hearts need minerals to function properly. If a person gets severely depleted of minerals, he can experience cardiac arrest. Extended water fasting can also lead to kidney damage. As toxins rush out of the body, the kidneys can experience toxic overload. Enemas or herbs that move the colon can help transport the rush of toxins out of the body and may reduce damage to essential organs—but this does not eliminate the concern.

Water fasting has proved beneficial for some people, but that does not mean it is good for everyone. Certain restrictive diets for extended periods in which a person is not consuming a variety of healthy foods or juices can lead to health issues. Dr. Foster said she has seen fruitarians, raw foodists, and others who were extreme in their eating habits for an extended time end up in the hospital because of protein deficiencies, fungal infections, and other illnesses. Though well meaning, their strict dietary choices resulted in more harm than good.

IF YOU CHOOSE TO WATER FAST...

If you decide to take on a water-only fast, plan to consume two quarts to a gallon of the purest water available every day of the fast. Although daily consumption of distilled water is not recommended due to its lack of minerals, it is a perfect choice for a water fast because it has the natural ability to bind to toxins.

Water fasts are challenging not only because you are not taking in any calories but also because of the uncomfortable symptoms of detoxification. Depending on how toxic you are at the start of your fast, you may experience more intense discomfort, especially if you haven't properly prepared your body for the fast. It can become difficult to continue on your own if the symptoms become too intense.

According to Dr. Joel Fuhrman, after water fasting for about two days for women and three days for men, the body goes into a state called *ketosis*.[3] This is a state in which the body begins to fuel itself by consuming fat cells. Because the length of time one can safely operate in ketosis varies from person to person, it may be wise to conduct this kind of fast under the supervision of a health professional. Such a professional can help you manage the discomfort of the detox symptoms as well as let you know when you've reached a state of "true hunger" and need to end the fast.

Consider a supervised fast

Let's discuss what a supervised water fast might look like. As I have already pointed out, water fasting can be dangerous—even fatal—without proper preparation and supervision. However, people who want to alleviate serious health conditions or diseases, such as cancer, multiple sclerosis, lupus, or fibromyalgia, might consider a supervised water-only fast.

Individuals who are extremely overweight and need to lose weight may also want to investigate the benefits of water fasting. Because there can be a connection between obesity and emotional issues, eating disorders, and addiction, a trained health professional would be a great partner for achieving the right outcome. Health professionals are well trained in knowing how to support behaviors that promote long-term healthy lifestyle changes and in discouraging behaviors that don't.

So how do you find the right health professional to supervise your water fast? On the International Association of Hygienic Physicians (IAHP) website (www.iahp.net), there is a listing of primary-care doctors who provide certified fasting supervision. You can search them by location to find a physician near you. Others offer supervision through their retreats or clinics. Though you would have to travel to their facility or venue away from home, this could be an added benefit, as you would have a chance to focus on your fast and your health goals without the distractions of your daily life. (You can always come to my retreats too, of course—though you would not be water fasting. I recommend juice fasting for my clients, which consists of consuming fresh juices that are chock-full of nutrients.)

Another option for those who cannot or prefer not to travel is phone consultations. Some of the IAHP physicians offer their clients remote guidance and supervision. However, they may extend this service only if you are in good health and do not have health issues that would require you to consult a doctor frequently during a fast.

Finally you can talk to your own primary-care doctor to see if she or he is available to monitor your health during your water-only fast. Just keep in mind that not all doctors are familiar with the unique things that can happen in a body during fasting. You can also look for a naturopathic doctor, holistic practitioner, or other alternative-medicine or natural-health professional.

Can you supervise yourself?

Many healthy people have completed water-only fasts successfully on their own. You know your body better than anyone, and if you are in good health, have a solid plan, and have properly prepared your body for rapid detoxification with other types of fasts such as juice fasting first, then you may be able to self-supervise your water fast.

Here are some tips for self-supervising a water fast:

+ **Start small.** If you've never water-fasted before, start with a short, one-day, regular (non-water) fast such as those I have previously described. Or try intermittent fasting (see chapter 2 for more information) or fasting from one meal a day. Don't bite off more than you can chew, such as attempting a ten-day fast. Instead take it slow.

+ **Try cleansing.** If you have poor eating habits, do a cleansing diet for one or two weeks first—maybe even a month or more—before trying a water fast. I recommend you join my thirty-day detox challenge.

+ **Take it up a notch.** Once your body has been properly nourished and cleansed and has some experience with detoxification and its symptoms, you could try an occasional one-day water fast.

+ **Get plenty of rest.** Your body is working hard to cleanse, purify, and heal itself during a water fast, and it will need lots of rest. Also remember that during a water fast you are not consuming any calories and your energy may be low. Nap when you need to. Pay attention. Listen to your body, and be ready to give it the rest it needs.

+ **Research.** Learn for yourself the pros and cons of water fasting in intervals and for various lengths of time.

+ **Above all, listen to your body.** Be ready to respond to any of your body's needs during your fast.

Additional considerations

With water-only fasts you will tend to lose weight rapidly because you will be shedding mostly water weight at first. After completing the fast, you will put some of the weight back on just as quickly as it came off. Most people report losing an average of one pound every day of their fast.[4] This kind of weight loss usually accompanies longer-term fasts. But do keep in mind that longer-term water-only fasts may need to be monitored carefully to avoid physiological complications.

As I stated above, listen to your body, and give it the rest it needs during this kind of fast. You may find that you need to slow down from your normal activities, avoid driving, or steer clear of emotional or frustrating situations. This need for rest can vary from person to person, often depending on one's body weight; overweight individuals may feel more energetic, and thinner individuals may feel more tired because their body is working to save energy. You may even find that light exercise, such as walking or stretching, is too much for you. The key again is to listen to your body.

To add another layer of detox benefits to your water fast, consider adding dry-skin brushing to your routine as well as deep-breathing exercises. These two practices will increase your body's ability to release toxins through the skin and airways. You will also want to make sure your bowels are moving every day. Add psyllium powder to your water— usually 1 to 2 tablespoons in 8 ounces of water. (Always follow the directions on the product you purchase.) It will act as a natural laxative to help toxins move out of your body.

As you come to the end of your fast, it is important to work your way back to eating solid foods very carefully. Start by drinking fresh vegetable juices and slowly eating juicy fruits, such as watermelon—in very small pieces at first. You could also add a green smoothie for dinner. Starting right back in with eating steak or hamburgers has had fatal results for some people. Being under supervision would be helpful in breaking a water-only fast properly, especially a water fast that is longer than a few days.

See the frequently asked questions in chapter 6 for a list of foods you can eat as you come off a fast and the order in which you should reintroduce them into your daily diet.

Your Body Needs Water

Getting plenty of pure water is important at all times. But when you fast, it's imperative! The average adult body is between 60 and 65 percent water, and the brain is made up of about 75 percent water. If you fail to hydrate your body well, you can do damage as you fast because you won't be flushing away toxins that get released from fat cells. Drink up! This will also give you energy.

Burn Fat and Flush out Coxins

Your body will not function properly without adequate water to carry out its everyday processes. In fact, your body needs pure water more than it needs daily food, as you can go without food much longer than you can without water.

Water also plays a significant role when it comes to achieving and maintaining a healthy weight. Drinking the right amount of water increases the rate at which your liver metabolizes fat. And what many people may not realize is that drinking an adequate amount of water every day reduces water retention. When you don't drink enough water, your body holds on to water.

As an advocate of fresh juice, I will point out that while juice has an abundance of water and is one of the most desirable beverages for health and weight loss, it is a food and as such does not take the place of water. So in addition to freshly made juice, you also need to drink at least eight glasses of water a day.

Do you know that many times when you feel hungry, your brain is

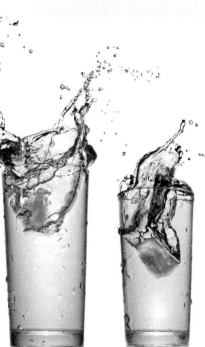

actually sending you a signal that your body needs water? Oftentimes we eat food when we should be drinking water instead. So try this the next time you feel hungry: drink a glass of water and wait fifteen minutes. Chances are, your feelings of hunger will pass.

In his book *Your Body's Many Cries for Water* Dr. F. Batmanghelidj says that overweight people often "don't know when they are thirsty; they also don't know the difference between 'fluids' and 'water.'"[5] He goes on to share the stories of several people who lost more than thirty pounds just by exchanging water for their favorite beverage.

Additionally, when you drink a glass

of water twenty to thirty minutes before a meal, you are likely to eat less. In her research Dr. Brenda Davy, associate professor of human nutrition, foods, and exercise at Virginia Tech, reported that "people who drank two glasses of water 20 to 30 minutes before every meal lost weight more quickly initially and lost significantly more weight long term than those who didn't." She also discovered that "people who drank water before meals ate an average of 75 fewer calories at that meal."[6]

Those 75 calories are significant when you add them all up. If you eat the standard three meals a day and 3,500 calories equal one pound, you could lose about twenty pounds in one year just by drinking more water!

Give your metabolism a boost

Though you may be aware how important a high metabolism is, it is good to fully understand what it does and how it can be slowed down, causing you to gain weight. Metabolism is the process by which your body uses food and water for energy to sustain your life. If your body is not quickly using what you put in it, the unused fuel can start to hang around and turn to fat. Increasing your body's use of the food and water you put in it can prevent fat formation, and it can also help you lose weight.

The liver is an organ in the body that carries out many functions, including fat metabolism. When the kidneys are overworked, which happens when they do not have enough water to do their work, the liver will do some of the work for them. When this happens, liver productivity is diminished, which decreases fat metabolism. When you drink the right amount of water every day, the kidneys can do their job, which allows the liver to focus on its primary functions.

Studies show that drinking 500 ml of water can help increase metabolism by as much as 30 percent![7] Similarly, being just 1 percent dehydrated can cause a drop in metabolism.[8] So raise your water glass throughout the day, and drink to a vibrantly healthy body!

How Water Helps You Fast

- Suppresses the appetite
- Improves digestion
- Energizes the body
- Helps prevent water retention and bloating
- Reduces cholesterol
- Helps tone muscles
- Flushes toxins from the body
- Stops the hunger-vs-thirst confusion

Get energized

One of the major secrets of water lies in the energy bonds formed between its hydrogen and oxygen atoms. The relatively weak hydrogen-bond length of H_2O molecules, for example, affects the electrostatic forces around them in a way that changes the energy of electrons in your RNA. RNA, the carrier molecule, transmits DNA information into cells, controlling their chemical reactions.[9]

This means one thing for you: energy! And when you fast, you need all the energy you can get.

Each of your cells produces energy fuel in the mitochondria known as ATP, and water is a part of that energy production. Without energy fuel you feel like being a total couch potato all day long. When your cells are fired up, you feel like getting things done, exercising, choosing the stairs rather than the elevator, and taking a few extra steps to get to your car, which you parked a distance away for exercise purposes.

THE CASE FOR PURIFIED WATER

Water has an amazing story that science is only beginning to discover. However, our lack of knowledge has led us to take water for granted. We abuse it, pollute it, and forget how vital it is to our health. When we go digging through the earth looking for oil and natural gas using a process called fracking, we inject thousands of gallons of toxic chemicals into our ground, which pollutes our water supply. As we learn more about the hidden mysteries of this precious element that quantum physicists are just beginning to unravel, it would be wise for us to think twice about how we use our limited natural resources.

In most areas of our country, tap water (and bottled water that originates from tap water) is loaded with fluoride and other chemicals. Though you may have heard that fluoride is vital to your dental health, the exact opposite is true. In a small town in India where rock erosion and volcanic activity increase the amount of fluoride in the drinking water, a group of researchers studied the recurring health problems of the people who live in the town and drink the water. What they discovered is that fluoride is anything but a cavity fighter.[10] It is a toxin that leads to tooth decay, weakened immunity, thyroid disorders due to displaced iodine, and accelerated aging due to cell damage. And fluoride is just one of the many detrimental chemicals added to our water every day.

For all these reasons I recommend that you get a good water purifier—unless you have pure well water that has been tested for contaminants and is free of them. I recommend either a ceramic filter or a distiller. Whatever machine you choose, make sure you get one that removes most of the fluoride—and not many of them do because it's difficult to get rid of. Though I do not recommend distilled water on a regular basis, it does help you detox when fasting.

HOW MUCH WATER SHOULD YOU DRINK?

Perhaps you are one who waits until your mouth is dry to drink some water. If so, you have waited too long! By the time you feel thirsty, you are already very dehydrated. Don't wait until your mouth feels like a cotton ball; drink water throughout the day. How much water? Let's see.

To determine the amount of water a person needs, some experts came up with a simple equation: your weight divided by two equals the number of ounces of water you should drink each day. If you weigh 200 pounds or more, you should drink about 100 ounces, or nearly one gallon, of water each day.

If you discover that the number of ounces you need to drink is far more than what you are currently drinking, start with drinking eight glasses of water a day and work up to your needed number of ounces for your weight. After a week you should be used to drinking the amount of water you need.

FLAVOR TO THE RESCUE

Many people won't drink water because they don't like the way it tastes. (If you get a water purifier, you might start to like it.)

Rather than not drink water at all, get creative. Try adding natural flavor to your water. Lemon water, lemon-ginger water, cucumber water, mint water, or cranberry water (flavored with a splash of pure unsweetened cranberry juice) are all refreshing and healthy ways to make water more pleasing to your taste buds. Maybe you've had water like this at your favorite spa. Well, you can make it for yourself at home. Plus you'll get an added bonus: lemon, cranberry, and cucumber are all natural diuretics, which means they help flush undesirable waste and toxins out of the body and eliminate water weight. Drink several glasses of lemon, cranberry, or cucumber water when beginning your fast because the body always eliminates water before body fat. This will help you feel more energized as you get rid of toxins.

Keep in mind, though, that when water is flavored—even naturally—it loses some of the cleansing purposes that are absolutely key for weight loss and health. Water is an information carrier, and as soon as there is something in it, it takes on another message. It is now received in the body as food. So even if you don't like plain water, try your best to drink several glasses of pure water each day.

You can also start your day with a cup of hot water and lemon with a pinch of cayenne pepper. This helps get your liver moving in the morning, which is important for metabolizing fat and helping your liver flush toxins.

Here are a couple of creative water recipes to boost the flavor in your water and deliver additional health benefits to your body:

Snappy Water

1 handful fresh mint
½ cucumber, sliced
1 Tbsp. grated fresh ginger
1 lemon, sliced

Place all ingredients in a pitcher, and fill to the top with pure water. Place it in the refrigerator. In a few hours, you will have "Snappy Water"—a delicious alternative to store-bought flavored waters.

Sun Water

Have you ever made sun tea? The idea of sun water is somewhat the same, but without the tea bags. Fill your glass container with purified water, and place it outside for the day. You will have vitamin D–infused water by day's end.[11]

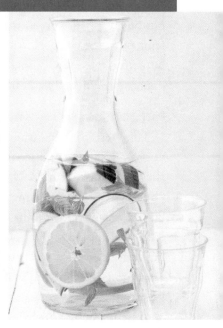

OTHER BEVERAGES YOU CAN DRINK WHILE FASTING

Green tea, herbal tea, and coconut water are other cleansing beverages you can drink during a fast. These beverages are not included for water fasting, but for all other fasts they are great additions.

Green tea

Rich in antioxidants, the phytonutrient catechins, and other polyphenols, green tea helps protect you against inflammation, cancer, and other ailments. It is especially useful in helping you shed unwanted weight by acting thermogenically to rev up your metabolism. Thermogenesis is the process by which heat is produced in the body. Much of the thermogenic action in green tea is due to epigallocatechin gallate (EGCG), a potent polyphenol. EGCG also appears to increase the effectiveness of weight-loss supplements, such as 5-HTP and tyrosine.

As you can see, green tea is a great beverage to make part of your daily meal plan. To experience the benefits listed above, drink at least one cup of organic green tea made with purified water every day. With about one-third of the caffeine found in a cup of coffee, it's a good choice, but be aware that green tea may irritate you if you are sensitive to caffeine or have low adrenal function. White tea has less caffeine and may be better tolerated. Actually white tea has the same types of antioxidants as green tea but in higher quantity.

Herbal tea

Time-tested herbal tea recipes have been passed down through generations of Chinese and Japanese people and many other cultures around the world for centuries. Dandelion and nettle teas are very detoxifying. Ginger tea is anti-inflammatory and has many other medicinal benefits. If weight loss is your goal, look for slimming herbal teas at your local health-food store. You may also enjoy hibiscus herbal iced tea. It's one of my favorites and acts as an anti-inflammatory. (I like Traditional Medicinals' organic hibiscus, which also has blackberry leaf and lemongrass leaf.)

When choosing green, white, and herbal teas, look for those that are organically grown. Also, unbleached tea bags are better than bleached.

Coconut water

Lastly, as one of the highest natural sources of electrolytes known to man, coconut water is an excellent drink option when you've been sweating profusely in a sauna or after you complete a workout. It's a good electrolyte replacer. In some remote areas of the world coconut juice is even administered intravenously for short-term purposes in emergency hydration situations.[12] Be aware, though, that coconut water does contain carbs, so limit your consumption to no more than one serving per day if you are watching your weight or you have a challenge with carbs.

SAY NO TO THESE BEVERAGES WHILE FASTING

While you are fasting, it is imperative that you carefully monitor what goes in your body. If you have everyday routines of drinking coffee or tea in the morning, a meal-replacement shake or soda at lunch, and a glass of wine to end the day, you will need to make some adjustments during this time. All of those drinks impact your body's ability to detox and maintain health.

Let's take a closer look, starting with coffee and tea.

Coffee and black tea

Two of America's favorite hot drinks, coffee and black tea, are very acidic and quite dehydrating—and remember what I said earlier about how dehydration interferes with weight loss? For every cup of coffee or black tea you drink, you need two to three glasses of pure water to neutralize the acid these drinks create in your body. High levels of acid cause your body to hang on to fat and not let it go just to protect your vital organs. Your body will even make more fat cells if it doesn't have enough storage cells for the acids. The acids also affect your joints and can contribute to your experiencing pain.

Though the ultimate health goal would be to omit coffee and black tea entirely, start by limiting your intake to just one cup of either drink per day. This will help lower the acidity in your body. You can also cut back by watering it down until you let it go. However, I highly recommend that you exchange coffee or black tea for green tea, which has one-third less caffeine than coffee and is more alkaline.

Soft drinks

Soft drinks are another type of beverage I recommend people avoid at all costs. If you have any form of rheumatism, arthritis, fibromyalgia, weight issues, cellulite, stiffness, aches and pains, or any disease—and if you simply want to remain healthy—then you cannot afford to drink any soft drinks. Not only are they very acidic, but they are also loaded with toxins. As long as you drink any kind of soda, you'll find it very difficult to lose weight and achieve great health. In fact, you may continue to gain weight.

Soft drinks are also loaded with phosphorus, which leaches calcium from bones. You could end up with severe osteoporosis and crippled for life.

Advertisers sometimes appear to be encouraging a more healthy lifestyle choice by recommending that consumers substitute diet soda for the more sugary versions. However, their advertising claims are false. Diet soda has been proved to be even more fattening than regular soda.

In 2013 the *American Journal of Clinical Nutrition* published a four-teen-year study of more than 65,000 women who were regular soda drinkers.[13] The results were astonishing.

The study revealed that diet sodas actually "raised the risk of dia-betes more than sugar-sweetened sodas," regardless of the women's body weight. (We tend to relate diabetes directly to obesity. This is not quite the case when it comes to consuming diet sodas.) Further anal-ysis revealed that "women who drank one 12-ounce diet soda had a 33 percent increased risk of Type 2 diabetes," and women who drank one 20-ounce soda doubled that risk. And because of the addictive nature of the artificial sweeteners in diet sodas, the women who drank diet sodas drank twice as much soda as those who drank sugar-sweetened sodas.[14]

In light of disturbing statistics such as these, I highly recommend that you replace any soft drinks in your diet with water, lemon water, or cranberry water. You can make your own fizzes with sparking water and a splash of your favorite fruit juice. Your good choices in this small area will reward you with big results health-wise.

As you begin to eliminate soda from your diet, you may face with-drawal symptoms. This is simply because your body has become addicted to sugar—but that does not mean your body needs it. It's quite the opposite. Detox symptoms are harmless and will go away quickly. Stay with it, and you will see your vibrant health return.

For more information on how to break the sugar habit, read my book *The Juice Lady's Sugar Knockout*.

Vitamin water

Among the biggest scams soda manufacturers have conjured up is vitamin water, another drink you should avoid. The marketers of this supposedly healthy drink are taking advantage of the public's interest in health by adding the word *vitamin* to its name. They want you to believe that somehow this drink measures up to the nutrients in food. It doesn't even come close. And what's worse is that it is full of added toxins. Search the label, and you'll find health-harming additives such as high-fructose corn syrup—a primary cause of obesity, metabolic syn-drome, and diabetes. You will also find a list of food dyes that can ruin your health. Do yourself a favor and just choose pure water or home-made flavored water.

Sports drinks

Sports and electrolyte drinks contain brominated vegetable oil. Bromine is a halogen that interferes with iodine absorption and wreaks havoc on the thyroid. These drinks are also very acidic.

Many sports drinks contain as much as two-thirds the sugar of sodas. They also typically contain high-fructose corn syrup (which scars the liver), artificial flavors, and food coloring. None of these ingredients contribute to good health. Most of these drinks also contain high amounts of sodium (processed salt). And if they say "sugar free," that means they contain artificial sweeteners, which are even worse than high-fructose corn syrup.

Meal-replacement drinks

Popular in the traditional weight-loss market, meal-replacement drinks are made of mostly sugar and water. Other top ingredients for some of the more visible brands include corn syrup, maltodextrin (sugar), and fortified vitamins and minerals. Always read labels carefully before choosing meal-replacement drinks. It is far better to make your own with a quality protein powder and a plant milk with a little fruit blended in. Choose any of my smoothie recipes for a delicious meal-replacement shake.

Alcohol

There are many reasons to avoid wine, beer, and hard liquor, but I'll bet you haven't heard this one: alcohol will suppress the secretion of the hormone vasopressin (also known as ADH) from the pituitary gland.[15] Lack of vasopressin will cause general dehydration—even in your brain cells.

Habitual use of alcohol (and caffeine) will produce severe dehydration and can lead to inflammation, which can cause conditions such as arthritis, heart disease, and cancer. If you do occasionally indulge, drink two glasses of water after drinking an alcoholic beverage. But while you fast, alcohol is completely off the list, no matter what fast you choose.

By now you know the importance of hydration for energy. Ask yourself as you fast if you can really afford that wine or beer you may have become accustomed to drinking in the evenings. Giving it up is well worth it.

REVIVE AND RESTORE

One of the fastest ways to revive your body and renew your energy is to drink plenty of water. To keep track of how much you need to drink, measure out your water for the day. If you are water fasting, this is the key element of your day.

It may seem as though we have discussed a lot of dos and don'ts concerning water and other beverages, but as you incorporate these tips into your periodic fasting and detox routines, you will find that the health and energy you experience will cause you not to miss the harmful substances you once thought you couldn't live without. Liquid-only fasts provide one of the best ways to break poor eating habits and find your way to lasting health—body, mind, and spirit.

Chapter 4

YOU NEED TO DETOX

*It is only when we are empty that we
can start to think again.*
—PETER SEEWALD

WHILE YOU'RE ON your fasting journey, why not cleanse your body? This is the perfect time to think about detoxing. After all, you're eating less—maybe very little. But even if you're doing the Daniel fast, which allows for more food, this is a great time for a detox. The toxins will start jumping out of their hiding places as you eat less and as you avoid animal proteins, coffee, alcohol, sugar, and junk food. Now is the time to get rid of the toxic bad guys in style.

Think about your body as if it were your car. What if you never changed your oil or filters? You get one body to take you through life. You can get a new car engine but not a new body. To keep your body humming along like a well-maintained vehicle, you need to periodically cleanse your colon, liver, gallbladder, kidneys, lungs, lymphatic system, skin, and blood. These are your filter systems and organs of elimination.

The world outside our bodies is highly polluted, and when we make bad food choices in addition to being exposed to a toxic environment, we compromise the body's ability to perform its normal detoxing and elimination processes. Our bodies get overwhelmed by the toxicity levels that bombard them from the outside as well as the inside. As they work to protect us from toxic substances, elements such as mucus, toxins, and congestion get trapped in our fat cells and tissue spaces. The body reacts as if it is in a life-or-death battle and hangs on to those fat cells to save our lives. This means that we may not actually be able to shed excess weight, find healing, and achieve vibrant health without first cleansing our bodies.

Many health experts believe the average person has between five and twenty pounds of toxins accumulated in their bodies. Can you imagine? That's five to twenty pounds we could really feel great about dropping! As I mentioned before, researchers also found more than two hundred chemicals in the blood of newborn babies. Of particular concern to the researchers were "contaminants, including the controversial plastics additive bisphenol A, or BPA, which mimics estrogen and has been shown to cause developmental problems and precancerous growth in animals."[1]

When toxic substances accumulate in the body, diseases such as cancer can occur. These substances enter our bodies and weaken our systems and the organs that handle elimination. And as I mentioned, this toxic overload will lead to a slow metabolism and difficulty losing weight. Though you may find ways to successfully complete a very strict fad-diet program, losing some weight, the toxicity levels in your body will cause the weight to come right back.

A SOUPY, TOXIC MESS

Chemicals, pesticides, drug residues, heavy metals, and food additives are just some of the many toxins we encounter regularly. There is hardly a place we can go these days without being introduced to some form of toxin. Our environment and unhealthy food choices hit us with a one-two toxic punch. Internally our bodies are at war with endotoxins (toxins that exist inside the body), yeasts, fungus, and parasites that build up in our bodies like the sludge inside old pipes. If we do not cleanse the inside of our bodies regularly through detox and fasting, endotoxins build up in our liver, kidneys, and large and small intestines as impacted waste. They even build up in the mucous lining of our lungs and sinuses. When these toxins permeate brain tissue, they can contribute to things such as brain fog, emotional outbursts, and other neurological and psychological issues. They can also lead to serious problems such as dementia and Alzheimer's disease. Not even our skin and bones can escape the effects of toxic overload.

Considering that every organ in the body is burdened with this toxic soup, it is no wonder that our immune responses are compromised and we find ourselves sick, weak, in pain, unable to fight off infections, and looking older than we are. This is why we must take periodic fasting and cleansing seriously and make it a part of a healthy lifestyle.

Since World War II more than eighty thousand chemicals have been invented, and many of them have been widely dispersed into our environment. According to researchers, "Over 4 billion pounds of toxic chemicals are released by industry into the nation's environment each year, including 72 million pounds of recognized carcinogens. Of the top 20 chemicals discharged to the environment, nearly 75% are known or suspected to be toxic to the developing human brain."[2] Is it any wonder I recommend regularly detoxifying the body from head to toe?

Mom, Watch Out

It was determined by a study done by the University of California–San Francisco that almost every pregnant woman in the United States has various kinds of toxic environmental chemicals in her body—even some that have been banned for years.[3] Though this data isn't totally surprising due to our access to information about the harmful chemicals in our environment, it confirms that pregnant women in particular, or women who want to become pregnant, should be mindful of the potential toxic burden they carry. If they can go through a total-body detox before conceiving, the cleansing may help them reduce the risk of their babies suffering from birth defects and other health issues related to high toxicity levels in their [the mothers'] bodies.

TOXIC HIDE-AND-SEEK: NOW YOU SEE THEM

How do we get rid of these harmful substances we can't even see? Detox. That's the only way. So here's the question for you: If not now, then when?

The longer you go without detoxing your body, the more toxic waste backs up, causing your organs and systems of elimination to get behind in their work. The buildup starts in the intestines, with mucus and putrefaction clinging to the walls of the intestinal tract. This keeps nutrients from being properly absorbed, and poisons are routed back into the bloodstream.

When the liver is overwhelmed and congested, blood is not purified well, and toxins are let into the bloodstream. Stones may also form in the gallbladder and even the liver. In the kidneys, the body's filtration system, waste that is usually eliminated through the urine is sometimes recirculated through the body because the kidneys can't keep up with the amount of purification that is needed when the body is overburdened with toxins.

This is when we find our bodies beginning to tell us what's happening inside. We develop rashes, acne, eczema, or psoriasis, plus headaches, frequent colds and flu, tiredness, poor sleep—on and on it goes. These are the outward signs that our bodies can no longer deal with excess waste.

Your metabolism is next on the list of body functions that become encumbered by high toxicity levels. In order to protect itself, the body treats the toxins like the acids they are and tries to hide them away in fat cells. But they can't hide there forever. As part of this protective measure, the body will hold on to the fat cells, which leads to a slow metabolism and excess weight that is hard to lose.

One outward sign of toxins being stored in fat cells is cellulite—the lumpy, bumpy skin that sticks on our thighs like globs of cottage cheese. Additionally we begin to face clogged pores and issues with the lungs and the lymphatic system. Certain diseases that form in any of these areas are the most devastating signs of toxic overload.

I want to help you avoid getting to this point. If you are already dealing with a disease or disorder resulting from toxic overload, I want to help you find your way to optimal health.

All Her Cellulite Is Gone!

"This is the third week for me [on the thirty-day detox program]. I was so happy to look in the mirror and see all the cellulite in the back area gone! The skin is as smooth and toned as could be, without having worked out since we started. Wow, just wow! Keep up the work, everyone. It's so worth it. Also, I am not weighing till Monday, but I can tell I've lost a lot." —Julie

THESE KINDS OF DIMPLES AREN'T SO CUTE

You may have come to terms already with the fact that cellulite is not like any other fat. You've probably tried all kinds of creams, tonics, and exercises to rid yourself of it, only to find that it won't leave. Most commonly found on the thighs, hips, and buttocks, cellulite is made up of irregular fat deposits that are trapped within connective tissues and are full of fluid, toxins, lymph, and waste.

I hate to be the bearer of bad news, but I have to tell you: with all your attempts to work out like crazy and suffer through strict diets to get rid of this clingy goo, it will still be around even if you get to a size 0. As long as you have poorly functioning blood vessels, constipation, poor lymphatic drainage, and toxicity, cellulite is there to stay.

Toxins and fluids build up quickly when blood flow in the vessels is weak and slow. This causes difficulty for the body when it is time to expel fat from those areas. When waste elimination is not functioning well, toxins are not moved out of the body and end up being reabsorbed into organs such as the liver and kidneys, affecting the efficiency of the lymphatic system.

One way to get toxins pumped out of the body is through exercise. Other ways to get the lymph moving that I've found helpful are lymphatic drainage massage, an herbal tincture, and a machine called the lymphasizer. I have included the details for these treatments in the Resources appendix.

The processed and refined foods we eat—sugar, refined salt, caffeine, alcohol, tobacco, unhealthy fats and oils, refined carbohydrates, junk food, and fast food—also tax our lymphatic and circulatory systems, making it harder for our bodies to get rid of waste and easier for fat to be retained as cellulite. According to some experts, toxins are the main contributors to fat's being collected in those lumpy pockets in the first place.[4]

Even though exercise helps move toxins out of the body, it does not get rid of cellulite. Topical treatments such as creams, lotions, or massage may be of some benefit, but they will not smooth out all the lumps. Cellulite will not disappear until you detoxify your whole body, zeroing in on the colon and liver to improve elimination, circulation, and your metabolism. Once you get your lymph back in gear and begin to nourish your body with living foods and juices, you will notice that your metabolism gets a lively jolt. When all systems begin to function at higher levels, you will raise the odds of those bulges and bumps melting away.

I know from personal experience that the combination of a healthy diet and regular detoxing is the ticket to smooth, cellulite-free skin. The toxins are what create that undesirable cottage-cheese look in the first place. So flush out those toxins with your fast, and give yourself a smoother finish.

As you detox and toxins begin to move out of your body, it is important to include things such as massage to nourish, condition, and strengthen the once-sluggish blood vessels, further improving circulation. Then fat can be used as energy instead of stored as extra weight.

Your thighs don't have to continue to look like a pitted golf ball. Your commitment to a cleansing program will have you looking trimmer and sleeker before you know it—and you'll be healthy on the inside too!

Pesky Pesticides Add to the Pudge

Kaveh Ashrafi, MD, PhD, and a group of scientists from South Korea studied rats and observed that a common herbicide called atrazine caused the rats to gain excess weight, even though their feeding times and serving sizes remained the same. Ashrafi concluded that the "genes that play a role in reading signals on the way from the brain to the periphery to regulate fat are being acted upon by pesticides and all these things that are in the environment."[5]

In another study, this time with mice, the researchers exposed in utero mice to diethylstilbestrol (DES) for five days. DES is an estrogen-like drug once used to prevent miscarriage.[6] As a result of their exposure to this chemical, the mice fetuses were born at a normal weight and grew at a normal rate but ended up much fatter over time. As with the rat study, the mice were fed at normal times and with normal serving sizes. They also maintained a level of physical activity consistent with the mice that were not exposed to DES.

With DES now being used in livestock and poultry feed, the next logical conclusion is that this drug is showing up in our food and causing many of us who consume commercial animal products to gain weight. Dr. Ashrafi seems to agree: "Maybe environmental toxins are essentially drugs that we are taking without knowing it—and they're acting in this process to promote fat regulation."[7]

TOXIC PLASTIC AND EVEN MORE SERIOUS CONCERNS

What once was the whistle-blowing efforts of a few natural health professionals and groups has now become a well-covered story in mainstream health news. I'm talking about the harmful effects of consuming foods and beverages out of plastic containers. We are now well aware that plastic is made from chemicals that alter the body's natural hormone and endocrine functions. One such chemical, bisphenol A (BPA), commonly connected to a higher risk of cancer, premature puberty, heart disease, and more, is now being banned from many plastic containers. When you shop for new cups, water bottles, or food-storage containers, you may have noticed the advertisements boasting the product is BPA-free.

Though this could be considered a step in the right direction, *BPA-free* does not mean all the toxic contaminants have been erased from the plastic. In his article "Nine Health Risks That Aren't Worth Taking" Dr. Joseph Mercola points out that the chemicals that play a role in disrupting the gender hormones, such as estrogen and testosterone, are still left intact in many of the plastics we use every day. He reports: "*GreenMedInfo* wrote a nice review on this recently, revealing that many manufacturers the globe over have been switching to the equally toxic bisphenol known as Bisphenol S (BPS) in order to evade impending regulatory oversight, as well as to ride the 'BPA-free' marketing gravy train by misleading the consumer into thinking their products are bisphenol free, which they are not."[8] Yikes!

These harmful toxins leach into our food and drink just by our use of them. But what's worse is when we use them to heat up our leftovers in the microwave. Heat increases the rate at which our food absorbs these toxic properties. This is true even of the very popular BPA-free plastics.

I recommend that you don't subject your living foods to the nutrient-draining microwave. If you are going to reheat your healthy meats, fats, fruits, or veggies, reheat them in a stainless-steel or cast-iron pan on your stovetop or in the oven. It takes only a few minutes, and you won't be creating toxins in your food.

HOW TOXIC ARE YOU?

Do you have toxicity symptoms? You can take the toxicity quiz on my website to find out—or simply fill out the checklist below. (Go to http://www.juiceladycherie.com/Juice/toxic-take-the-quiz/ for the online version.)

Whether you score some points on the quiz or none at all, it is good for everyone to detox his or her body every year. Just as you don't wait until you have car problems before you get an oil change, you don't want to wait until your body is overwhelmed with toxins and sick before you implement a regular detoxification regimen. Our bodies are more valuable than our cars, and we should see detoxing as the body's oil-change process. You take your car in every three months or three thousand miles; you can treat your body to a regular detox at least once per year. Regular detoxing reduces symptoms and improves the health and vitality of all the systems in your body, helping you live longer and look younger.

Symptoms of Toxicity

- ❏ Acid reflux
- ❏ Arthritis
- ❏ Bloating
- ❏ Body aches and pains
- ❏ Cellulite
- ❏ Constipation
- ❏ Difficulty sleeping
- ❏ Dizziness
- ❏ Emotional and mental problems
- ❏ Excess weight
- ❏ Feelings of stress and anxiety
- ❏ Flatulence
- ❏ Headaches
- ❏ Hormone imbalances
- ❏ Inability to lose weight
- ❏ Indigestion
- ❏ Irritability
- ❏ Listlessness and fatigue
- ❏ Premature aging
- ❏ Restlessness
- ❏ Sinus problems
- ❏ Skin irritations or disorders
- ❏ Vision problems
- ❏ Weakness

She's Looking Great, Losing Weight, and Feeling More Energetic

"Yesterday was my last day of the Thirty-Day Detox Challenge, and I cannot tell you how great I feel! My body feels so clean! I have mental clarity and energy like no other. My skin is glowing. People who see me say, 'You look great.' I have had others ask my friends, 'What is she doing? She looks great!' I have lost weight. I didn't weigh before I started because my goal was not to lose weight as much as it was to detox. Weight loss is just a by-product of doing what is good for the body. I have to say I have lost fifteen pounds at least. I believe in detoxing the body, and your program has been awesome." —Anne

PREPARE FOR A FEW SYMPTOMS

The buildup of toxins in the body, as we just learned, leads to lots of unpleasant symptoms. But as you fast and cleanse, you may experience some other surprising symptoms. This is not unusual. Cleansing symptoms are part of the process for many people who fast and detox. You may not experience any of them, but if you do have a few, it's good to know about them in advance so you are not alarmed when something shows up. One young woman whom I was guiding through a detox got a rash during her cleansing process and ran to the emergency room to get a steroid shot. Doing something like this is quite counterproductive to the whole cleansing process. It adds more toxins into the body and prevents toxins from being expelled. Most toxic symptoms go away within a few days as the toxins are cleared from the system. It's important to assist your body in the elimination process rather than abruptly stopping the detox.

Here are some of the symptoms that may show up, especially during the first week or two of your fast:

- Abnormal perspiration
- Bloating
- Chills
- Cold hands and feet
- Constipation or diarrhea
- Elevated heart rate
- Fatigue
- Flu-like symptoms
- Headache
- Increased joint or muscle pain
- Itching, hives, or rash (sometimes assumed to be an allergic reaction)
- Low blood pressure
- Low-grade fever
- Nausea
- Swollen glands

Detox reactions—or the "healing crisis," as these symptoms are also called—occur as toxins are released and yeast and fungal organisms begin to die and leave the body. Sometimes, due to the nature of a detox fast, this elimination process happens at a rate the body wasn't quite ready for. But don't be alarmed. The symptoms do not last long. Make sure you help your body expel the toxins by drinking lots of water. Getting periodic enemas or colonics throughout your fast or detox will also help to reduce the flare-up of the detox reactions.

It's exciting to see how the body responds when we omit a host of unhealthy foods that drain our vitality. During a juice fast your body will purge toxins, especially if you haven't done much fasting or detoxing before. Usually the first two days are the most difficult because the toxins are being released. This is one reason I recommend Friday as a good day to start a fast. It's often the second and third days when you experience more toxins being released and thus more symptoms. You may experience a headache, nausea, diarrhea, a rash, itchy skin, halitosis, foggy brain, a spacey feeling, or tiredness. Or you may not experience much out of the ordinary. But if you do have a symptom or two, hang in there! You are detoxing. This too shall pass…literally. And you will feel so much better after your fast.

Dry brushing is another great tool to facilitate cleansing. Your skin is the largest organ of elimination. As you fast, your body will purge toxins through the skin. Get a natural-bristle brush and dry-brush before you shower. Start at your feet and move upward toward the heart. Then start at your wrists and move upward toward your shoulders and across your back.

The fast is also the time to quit coffee, alcohol, and/or smoking. To accomplish this with the least stress, reduce your use of these substances several days prior to beginning your fast. Going cold turkey can be a shock to your system, so start cutting back early.

DETOX YOUR WAY TO MORE ENERGY

As you make your way through your detoxification process, one of the first benefits you will experience is an amazing level of energy. With a highly toxic body and environment, your internal systems are used to running in slow motion. You may have gotten accustomed to the over-burdened, sluggish feeling caused by a buildup of waste and congestion. But all the energy being spent just to keep your body going with a heavy toxic load is going to be released, causing you to be more productive, clearheaded, and positive. All that sludge in your body will be moving out, freeing your systems to function at a higher level. You will begin to feel as if you can take on the world again!

Packed with energizing antioxidants, raw foods and juices are some of the best foods you can consume to gently detox. This is one reason I'm somewhat partial to the juice and/or smoothie fast. The antioxidants used in juices and smoothies attach themselves to the toxic substances in your body and carry them out. Without this overload your body doesn't have to carry a heavy weight around. How do you feel on a hike with a heavy backpack versus no backpack at all? Big difference, right? Without a backpack there's nothing but you, the path, and the fresh air. You might even be able to start jogging! That's what happens when your body starts to detox.

TIME TO GET TO WORK

So far we've discussed how toxic chemicals from the outside come into our bodies and interrupt and bog down the systemic functions on the inside, leading to all kinds of health issues—physical, mental, and some emotional. Now that we can see what problems are associated with accumulated toxic waste, it is time to get to work. Each of our organs connected to elimination needs to be cleansed so that our energy and vitality will be renewed, fat and cellulite lost, stubborn symptoms dissipated, and ailments, illnesses, and diseases healed. It's time to do a focused detox fast, which we'll cover in the next chapter.

My goal is to help you find your way to the glowing health and vibrancy that may have eluded you for years. By supporting your organs of elimination through cleansing and reconditioning, the built-in processes you currently have in your body for dealing with toxins, poisons, chemicals, yeasts, parasites, and internal by-products of metabolism will begin to function at an optimal level.

So what are you waiting for? Check out the next chapter on the detox fast, and let's get those toxins out of your system now.

Chapter 5

THE DETOX FAST

Fasting today makes the food good tomorrow.
—GERMAN PROVERB

F YOU ARE reading this chapter, you're probably interested in the detox part of a fast. There are people who will tell you that if you don't feel well when fasting, you're doing something wrong. Instead you are probably detoxing—and that's something very right. It's something we all need. This is spring cleaning for your body, soul, and spirit.

You have many options for general detoxing, from using a sauna, to ingesting herbs that help with detoxing, to drinking juices and eating a diet that are especially cleansing. You can also go after the real "bad boys" of the toxic world with heavy-metal detoxing. And finally, through a detox fast, you can focus in on the primary organs of elimination—the intestines, liver, and kidneys.

SPRING CLEANING FOR YOUR BODY AND SPIRIT

As we've discussed, fasting is a great time to be renewed, refreshed, and revitalized in your spirit. It is also a time to restart the systems in your body for optimal health and physical well-being and to bring restoration to your mind, body, and spirit. It is a lot like a threefold spring cleaning, in which mentally, physically, and spiritually you dive deep into the areas in your life that don't always get the attention they need and clean them up. With fasting you have a chance to hit the reset button; to rid yourself of toxic influences that hinder growth, clarity, and well-being; and to be refocused and recharged for your next season of life.

Completing specific detox programs aimed at purifying and cleaning up your blood and systems of elimination will enhance your fasting experience. In this chapter we will focus on cleanses for the intestines, liver, and kidneys, along with a few other detox recommendations that benefit the whole body.

When the toxic burden hanging over your major organs of elimination is removed, you'll find your ability to heal and be restored exponentially improved. I like to call this next series of detox protocols "spring cleaning," no matter the time of year, because you will get down deep into the cracks and crevices, folds and fissures of these specialized tissues and begin cleansing and repairing, rejuvenating and restoring, just as you would do in your home.

Are you ready? Let's get started!

Detoxification: How You Benefit

- A return of healthy bacteria and balanced intestinal flora
- Better sleep
- Clearer thinking and mental agility
- Curbed cravings for sugar, salt, junk food, alcohol, and nicotine
- Decongestion of mucus in the digestive and respiratory systems
- Higher levels of creativity
- Improved digestion

- Improved health and overall sense of well-being
- Loss of excess weight
- More energy
- Purified, freer-flowing blood
- Reduced joint and muscle pain
- Stabilized disposition and positive outlook
- Stronger immune system
- Vibrant, younger-looking skin

SPRING CLEANING FOR YOUR INTESTINES

Many of our nutrients are absorbed through the small intestine. Over the course of time our intestines get coated with plaque, and nutrient absorption becomes compromised. When we regularly consume overcooked, fried, spoiled, junk, or refined foods; cookies, candy, ice cream, alcohol, and coffee; and antibiotics and other prescription drugs, mucous secretion in the lining of our intestines is increased. For our bodies this is a normal immune response as the body attempts to protect itself against irritating foods. But over time this mucus begins to build up and form into a rubbery, plaque-like substance. The plaque becomes a hiding place and breeding ground for yeast overgrowth, specifically *Candida albicans*, as well as other parasites. For many years I had health problems as a result of parasites and candidiasis. It wasn't until I discovered the effectiveness of intestinal detoxification that I was able to witness the elimination of these kinds of rubbery substances from my body and find my way to complete health and healing.

Under normal circumstances our bodies are made to break down mucous secretions by producing pancreatic juices that help liquefy the mucus and move it along the digestive tract and out of the body. But when we are consuming the things I mentioned above on a regular basis, our digestive process becomes overwhelmed with all the mucus and cannot eliminate the overload of waste.

Our intestines become constipated when they are not able to move waste out of the digestive tract quickly. The longer the transit time (the time it takes for waste to move through the digestive tract and exit the body), the more waste has a chance to putrefy and ferment, forming gases and toxins that can be reabsorbed into the body. The longer our bodies are exposed to fermenting waste in our intestinal tracts, the greater the risk of developing diseases such as cancer.

Though you may have bought into the idea that one bowel movement a day is "regular," once a day is still not frequent enough to keep waste from putrefying in your system. If you eat three meals a day, you should have three bowl movements. Those having fewer bowel movements than meals are harboring a greater breeding ground for serious diseases and health issues. If that's the case for you, it's time to get this corrected.

Regularly cleansing your intestinal tract will help to ensure that toxins do not build up and overtax your elimination systems. You will also experience better nutrient absorption and overall improvement in digesting what you consume.

It's not hard to see why a clean intestinal tract is so important to good health. Please do check with your holistic doctor before beginning any detoxification program, especially if you have an intestinal disease such as Crohn's disease or diverticulitis.

Beginning your intestinal cleanse

A colon or intestinal cleanse is the best way to begin your detox program. You want your channel of elimination as clean as possible when your liver begins dumping toxins. You should create a detox regimen that includes a one-week colon cleanse two times per year. The first time you set out to cleanse your colon, you may need to plan for several weeks of cleansing in order to make sure all the plaque and waste that has built up over the years is thoroughly cleared out.

Here is a basic, daily to-do list to follow while cleansing your colon:

+ To jump-start your cleanse, I recommend that you go on a three- to five-day vegetable-juice fast. Begin each day with a cup of hot water and the juice of 1/4 lemon with a dash of cayenne pepper. This mixture will stimulate digestive juices and cause your bowels to loosen. It will also get the liver working.

+ Then stir 1 tablespoon of bentonite clay into a glass of water. Bentonite is an edible clay that forms a gel when combined with water and acts as a bulk laxative, binding toxins such as pesticides and transporting them out of the colon. To the bentonite clay and water add 1 tablespoon of fiber, such as ground flaxseeds, psyllium powder, and/or apple pectin. Mix it well with the bentonite clay and water, and drink the mixture right away, as it gels and will become too thick to drink if you wait. This will absorb water and expand in the colon, helping to remove toxins and mucus. After drinking the bentonite-fiber mixture, wait at least thirty minutes before eating. You should also drink this mixture before you go to bed and one to three times during the day.

- Make sure you drink at least eight glasses of purified water each day.

- Take an herbal cleansing product every day with dinner. Take it the first time the evening before you begin the cleanse. This will keep your intestinal tract moving. You should have two or three bowel movements each day. Look for a supplement that contains ingredients such as Chinese rhubarb root, barberry root, dandelion root, fringe tree root bark, arnia fruit, chebulic and belleric myrobalan fruit, meadowsweet aerial plant, English plantain, ginger root, fennel seed, peppermint leaf, fenugreek seed, and licorice root. (See the Resources appendix.)

- Take probiotics to replenish the good bacteria in the colon. You should follow the directions for your probiotic product. Most say you can take them with food, so you could take this at dinner along with the herbal cleansing product. If you need further help choosing the appropriate intestinal cleanse products, check out the Colon Cleanse Kit and the Internal Cleanse Kit (which comes with a free Colon Cleanse Kit) in the Resources section.

- Flush your intestinal tract by getting colonics or giving yourself enemas (see directions that follow) during your intestinal cleanse to assist in eliminating waste.

Note: If you take medications, bentonite clay should be consumed at least two hours before or two hours after you take your medication because it may interfere with absorption.

Two ways to flush your intestinal tract

There are two main ways to flush your intestinal tract when focusing on detoxing your intestines and colon, and those are colonics and enemas.

Colonics

Usually performed by a professional colon therapist, colonics or colon hydrotherapy involves gently pushing water into the colon to flush out built-up waste. It is a safe, drug-free process that uses purified, tempera-ture-regulated water to loosen and soften intestinal waste. I recommend getting one or two colonics per week during your colon cleanse. Not only helpful in removing excess waste, colonics can also be helpful in facilitating weight loss.

If this is the first time you are hearing of or considering colonics and you are thinking this is a far-out and borderline ridiculous health-nut idea, realize that some of the most successful and well-known people in the world take part in this process. From Hollywood royalty to the British royals themselves, celebrities know the advantages of regular colonics. Benefits such as reduced bloating and gas, brightened and whitened eyes, flattened bellies, weight loss, improved colon health, younger-looking and vibrant skin, and even shiny, voluminous hair have all been the result of colonics.

For my personal health I have combined colonics with juice fasting and intestinal herbal cleansing several times a year for more than fifteen years. On more than one occasion I experienced a two-pound weight loss after a colonic.

Having your colon irrigated brings much-needed hydration to the colon and assists in the removal of built-up fecal matter, mucus, and toxins. I understand that colonics can seem rather invasive and perhaps a bit embarrassing; however, in my experience, most practitioners work hard to make you feel at ease and will talk you through what to expect. As you are shopping for the right place to have this procedure done, look for a place that is clean and uses disposable tubes and hoses.

Enemas

If you are unable to locate a reputable colon therapist in your area, enemas are the next best thing. Like colonics, enemas provide a great way to restore regular bowel movements and to loosen and flush out intestinal debris that is released during a colon cleanse. Perhaps more commonly known than colonics, enemas have been used for centuries to improve or maintain bowel health.

An enema is something you can do yourself—no need to involve a colon therapist, as with the colonic. The process involves infusing water into your colon through your anus. With similar benefits to those you would experience with colonics, this process is the perfect companion to an intestinal cleanse. It is actually a good idea to do enemas as you cleanse. You'll experience fewer detox symptoms if you quickly get the toxins out of your body.

If you'd like to give it a try, here's what you will need to do:

+ Purchase an enema bag or bucket from your local drug-store or online. Usually the independent stores will be your best bet for finding them. Find the enema bags that look like hot-water bags. I actually prefer the bucket, and it's far less expensive. You will need to purchase that online.

+ Once you are home and ready to take the enema, fill the bag or bucket with one quart of warm filtered or distilled water.

+ Because you will begin with flushing the descending colon, which is on the left side of your body, it's best to lie down on your left side.

+ Tighten the clamp on the hose to avoid having water leak all over the floor; then insert the end of the hose into your anus.

+ Next, reach behind, locate the clamp, and release it to let the water run into your colon until you start to feel full. You can tighten the clamp for just a moment to allow the water to run deeper into the colon. Release the clamp again to let the rest of the water in the enema bag or bucket empty out into your colon.

+ Now relax and wait for a few minutes on your left side; then turn on your back for a couple of minutes to allow the water to go across your transverse colon. If this is your first enema, you may find it hard to wait for the full infusing process to complete. If this is the case, go to the toilet and evacuate all the fluid and waste. If you do have experience with enemas and can wait as the water infuses your entire colon, proceed to the next step.

• Turn onto your right side for a couple of minutes so the water can flow into the ascending colon. At this point you may feel that it is time to evacuate all the water and waste in the toilet. Take the time to make sure everything comes out. After this first bowl movement you will still need to stay close to the bathroom for another ten or fifteen minutes, just in case more waste needs to be released.

Though simple water enemas are the easiest to do and have great results, you can add other fluids to enhance the detoxification process. Try adding 1–2 ounces of organic wheatgrass juice to 2 cups of water. Combine it with the warm water for the enema to reach a total of one quart of liquid. Wheatgrass juice contains many healing nutrients, especially chlorophyll, which is a great detoxifier.

Some colon-cleansing protocols include coffee enemas, in which the caffeine in the coffee acts as a stimulant to the liver, causing it to release more toxins. If you do a coffee enema, make sure you use organic coffee.

These Newlyweds Discovered the Power of Colon Cleansing

"I wanted to give you a review of the colon cleanse to let you know how much you've changed my life and my husband's life!

"Our health journey started a little over three years ago, when we watched *Fat, Sick and Nearly Dead* together as a newly married couple. I had seen it by myself before, but for some reason it was the second time that motivated me to look into juicing for us. At the time I didn't think either my husband or I had any health problems, but I had the idea of getting more nutrition in our diets, and I wanted to see if juicing made us feel better in general.

"Around that time I mentioned to an acquaintance that I wanted to try juicing, and he told me to look up 'the Juice Lady.' After that I think I read three or four of your books in a row. By far, my favorite is *Juicing, Fasting, and Detoxing for Life*. I refer back to it regularly to this day. After reading *Juicing, Fasting, and Detoxing for Life*, all of a sudden I was looking at our bodies, health, and nutrition with new eyes.

"For one thing, I never seriously thought about what exactly goes on in the digestive system, what each of my organs does, or what various digestive symptoms actually mean. I never gave any real consideration to my bowel movements, even if they weren't regular or normal. I used to think that things such as bloating, constipation, diarrhea, and acid reflux were just symptoms that everybody got every so often. It never occurred to me that those are symptoms of digestive dysfunction as a result of what goes in the body.

"This led me to arrive at one big, real, overall revelation. I was already a Christian believer, but suddenly it dawned on me: God designed and created our bodies, so *of course* He designed and created foods that would nourish and fuel our bodies to function properly—optimally! And it hit me: all of those packaged and bottled foods in the middle aisles of the grocery store were *not* created by God but by men in laboratories. Of course it makes sense to eat natural, organic, whole foods that are found in nature because that's what God provided us from the very beginning. And that's what man ate until he started to mess with God's design by processing and manipulating natural ingredients to produce nutrient-depleted and even toxic 'foods' that God did not intend for us to consume.

"This revelation confirmed what I already knew, but in a totally new way: God's ways are perfect, and going against His design and plan only brings dysfunction, sickness, and pain. I used to think this way only in terms of moral decisions and spiritual health, but it is true for decisions we make regarding our physical health as well.

"Anyway, I started to pay attention to my digestion and my husband's, and I realized just how bad my husband's was. Once I made a list of all his symptoms, I realized they all pointed to a toxic colon and a toxic liver. Right around that time he also had his first bout ever with kidney stones. The diagnostic imaging not only revealed that he had numerous stones in his kidneys, but it also confirmed a fatty section on his liver as well (though the doctor reported the fatty section to be within 'normal' limits and did not show any concern!). Further testing revealed a high level of uric acid. All of this made perfect sense according to the symptoms of the various organ dysfunctions in your book.

"To try to make this long story short, I began juicing for us and made changes to our diet. I started gradually at first, but then a change in our circumstances allowed me to quit my job, and then I was really able to invest the time, energy, and research into making more significant changes for us. My husband's energy had improved, but he still had poor digestion. It seemed as if he was constantly vacillating between constipation and loose stools, and he was not having a bowel movement every day.

"I had us do a five-day juice fast. I had him get your Colon Cleanse Kit at the same time. During the cleanse he released a lot of mucoid plaque. Afterward he began to have at least one regular, healthy bowel movement every day. I can't tell you how relieved and thrilled I was! And still am. Over time his bowel movements increased to one or two BMs a day.

We are now doing a second colon cleanse for him (and a first for me). I am looking forward to improving our digestion even more.

"I could go on and give more examples of victories we've had with my husband's other symptoms, but this e-mail is already a lot longer than I planned. But I want to say thank you for your work, for your wisdom, and for changing our lives." —Andrea

SPRING CLEANING YOUR LIVER

William James said, "Is life worth living? It all depends on the liver." As the primary place for the body to store toxins it can't get rid of, the liver plays a vital role in the body's natural detoxification process. Every chemical you consume, from highly toxic pesticide and herbicide residues to medications and alcohol, passes through the liver. For some people it doesn't take much more than exposure to these toxic substances for their livers to become weakened, irritated, and unable to perform their proper function.

Some very commonly consumed products, such as Tylenol (acetaminophen), high-fructose corn syrup, and even agave syrup, which is also fructose, can scar or destroy liver cells in some people. Alcohol is another substance that contains toxins that harm the liver. Alcoholics are known to have a high risk for liver disease, especially liver cancer. For other people, consuming too much sugar can cause fatty liver. Fatty liver is in fact on the rise, even in younger people. We need to detox from sugar. For help and support in doing this, see my book *The Juice Lady's Sugar Knockout*.

As a result of our modern diet many people have considerable liver congestion and also stones. Even if a person does not have a history of gallstones, he may still be at risk of developing them because of how he eats. People who have had their gallbladders removed need to be especially mindful of caring for their livers. Stones and congestion in the liver are a big hindrance to achieving and maintaining good health. They are indeed one of the major reasons people become ill and have difficulty either recuperating from illness or reversing disease.

One reason people are being diagnosed with high cholesterol is that their livers are congested. This is true even for people who eat a very healthful diet and exercise regularly. Your liver creates more cholesterol than a normal diet contains. Even if you stopped eating all foods that contain cholesterol and reduced your intake to zero grams of cholesterol, your body would simply manufacture more. So if you notice that even with healthy eating and regular exercise your cholesterol is still high, a liver detox may be in order.

As stones grow and congestion increases, the pressure on the liver causes it to produce less bile, which is a substance that aids in removing cholesterol from the body. When less bile is produced and then excreted out of the body, a rise in cholesterol levels will occur. I have a thought: What if everyone diagnosed with high cholesterol were put on a liver cleanse before anything else? Cholesterol-lowering drugs are not the answer. They can actually cause harm to the body and add to its toxic load.

Because our health depends on an efficient and effective liver, it is important to keep it strong and nourished through regular cleansing and a liver-supporting diet. Cleansing your liver is one of the best things you can do to restore balance to your body. Taking a cholesterol-lowering drug will not get to the root of the problem.

Because conventional medicine has limited matrixes and methods to monitor the health of your liver, cleansing and detoxifying the liver on a regular basis is a necessary preventative measure. By the time your doctor's blood tests are able to pick up any abnormalities in the function of your liver, the damage has already been done. This is because liver cells have to rupture in order for their very strong enzymes to be indicated in blood tests. Usually people are at an advanced stage of liver-cell destruction, suffering from a disease such as hepatitis, before impaired function is discovered. Most people who have liver congestion, toxicity, or stagnation have perfectly normal levels of liver enzymes in their blood. Thus it takes many years before diagnosis of liver problems becomes possible.

Because we won't really benefit from a liver cleanse if the liver is full of parasites, I usually combine a parasite cleanse with a liver cleanse. With parasites in the way it is difficult to remove stones, congestion, or fat, and you may end up feeling sick. This is not the result we want. Getting rid of parasites with the liver cleanse yields the best results. (See the Resources appendix.)

Signs it may be time to detox your liver

The following symptoms sneak up on us, causing interruptions in our health and well-being:

+ Allergy and sinus issues

+ Anal itching (this can also be caused by parasites)

+ Bad breath

+ Body odor

+ Brown spots on the face and hands

+ Cellulite

+ Cherry angiomas (small smooth or raised red spots on the skin)

+ Coated tongue

+ Constipation

+ Dark circles under the eyes

+ Difficulty sleeping

+ Dizziness

+ Drowsiness after eating

+ Fatigue

+ Frequent urination at night

+ Gas and bloating resulting in belching and/or flatulence

+ Headaches or migraines

+ Hemorrhoids

+ Inability to tolerate heat or cold

+ Irritability

+ Low libido

+ Lower-back pain

+ Memory loss

+ Menstrual problems and PMS

+ Muscle or joint aches or pains

+ Nervousness and anxiety

+ Overall feeling of being unwell

+ Pain around the right shoulder blade and shoulder (also connected with gallbladder congestion)

+ Puffy eyes and/or face

+ Red nose

+ Sallow or jaundiced complexion

+ Stomach or intestinal pain and discomfort

+ Trouble with mental focus and concentration

+ Yeast overgrowth

When you begin to notice you are experiencing any of the symptoms on this list, it may be time for you to cleanse your liver.

Foods your liver will love

Your liver is working at its best when there are no obstacles preventing it from keeping your body toxin-free. But when it is overburdened by your overconsumption of dead foods and processed treats, it cannot do its job. A seven-day liver detox focuses on optimizing liver function by cleansing, protecting, and nourishing the liver. Living foods, juices made from them, and supplements such as those mentioned below that you consume for seven days will provide a nutrient-rich environment that will restore your liver.

Veggies that will support your liver cleanse

The following vegetables will help you cleanse and nourish your liver. Try to use organic veggies as much as possible so you are not introducing more pesticides and toxins while you are detoxing. And try to eat and juice the veggies on this list in abundance for the cleanse week:

+ Artichokes

+ Beets

+ Broccoli

+ Brussels sprouts

+ Cabbage

+ Carrots

+ Cauliflower

+ Celery

+ Chives

+ Cucumber

+ Eggplant

+ Garlic

+ Green beans

+ Kale

+ Kohlrabi

+ Lettuce

+ Mustard greens

+ Okra

+ Onion

+ Parsley

+ Parsnips

+ Peas

+ Pumpkin

+ Spinach

+ Squash

+ Sweet potatoes or yams

Cleansing Your Liver Will Make You a Whole New Person

When you cleanse your liver, you can expect a clearer, brighter complexion; the disappearance of dark circles under the eyes and age spots; improved digestion; easier weight loss and disappearance of cellulite; increased energy; and better, more restful sleep. If you were waking multiple times a night to go to the restroom, you should expect this issue to go away or at least improve. Your aches and pains, headaches, allergies, and puffiness in your face will all go away. You will be in a better, more stable mood. You will begin to feel a general sense of health and wellness, and your memory, mental clarity, and focus will spark up.

Supplements that will support your liver cleanse

The supplements on this list are included in my seven-day liver cleanse program as part of the Thirty-Day Detox Challenge; you can also find the program in my book *Juicing, Fasting, and Detoxing for Life*. This book includes recipes that provide great benefit for your liver. The morning citrus-ginger-olive-oil shake, cleansing beet salad, carrot salad, mineral broth, and a menu plan for the seven-day program can all be found there.

+ **Milk thistle.** Milk thistle, with its active ingredient sily-marin, which contains powerful antioxidant properties, helps to prevent damage to the liver caused by free radicals. It also helps to enhance overall liver function and inhibits factors that cause hepatic damage.

+ **Artichoke powder.** Cyranin, a chemical found in arti-choke, is a liver strengthener. It helps increase bile production and strengthens the bile duct so that it's better able to contract. It also helps to protect the cell walls of the liver from damage and scarring by giving them the nutrients that make them stronger. Artichoke powder also aids in breaking up and mobilizing fat stored in the liver, making it useful in the fight to lower cholesterol.

+ **Turmeric.** Curcumin is the primary chemical found in turmeric that helps cleanse the liver, purify the blood, stimulate the gallbladder for improved bile secretion, and promote good digestion and elimination.

+ **N-acetyl-L-cysteine (NAC).** Helping to provide optimum antioxidant protection from free radicals caused by environmental pollution, cigarette smoke, and alcohol, NAC is often prescribed by natural-health practitioners for their patients who have mercury or heavy-metal toxicity. NAC binds to these toxins and helps the body excrete them.

+ **L-methionine.** An amino acid that helps the liver create glutathione, L-methionine assists with raising glutathione levels, which, in turn, helps the liver perform its natural detoxification functions.

+ **Beet leaf and black radish.** Beet leaf, which helps to balance blood pH levels and stimulate bile excretion, and black radish, which supports heavy-metal detoxification, work with the liver's detoxification process as well as its carbohydrate and fat metabolism.

+ **Dandelion.** Dandelion, used for centuries as a favorite of natural-health practitioners, promotes bile secretion and the elimination of metabolic waste.

+ **Garlic.** Your liver loves garlic! It helps to catalyze liver enzymes and boost its natural filtration qualities. A little bit goes a long way with this powerful vegetable, as it contains high concentrations of allicin and selenium. Both are natural compounds that fortify liver cleansing.

Juices that will support your liver cleanse

A few juices will make all the difference with your liver cleanse.

+ **Beet juice.** Used in naturopathic medicine to cleanse and support the liver, beet juice is made by juicing the root and the leaves. You can also make beet salad with the leftover pulp. Beets are the stars in my seven-day liver-cleansing program.

+ **Carrot juice.** Carrot juice, made up of organic freshly juiced carrots, helps to stimulate and improve overall liver function. Use leftover pulp to make into a tasty detox salad.

+ **Dark, leafy-green juice.** High in plant chlorophyll, leafy greens are one of our most powerful allies in cleansing the liver. They literally suck up toxins from the bloodstream; neutralize heavy metals, chemicals, and pesticides; and halt the progression of hyphae—the long, branching structures of yeast and fungus that spread systemically throughout the body. Juiced, eaten raw, and lightly cooked, greens such as beet tops, arugula, dandelion greens, spinach, mustard greens, kale, chard, collards, kohlrabi leaves, and chicory offer a powerhouse of cleansing for the liver.

Foods to avoid while cleansing your liver

As you detox your liver, avoid foods that irritate the liver or produce an excess of mucus in the body, such as meat, dairy, sweets, alcohol, eggs, coffee, refined foods, soda pop, all oils and spreads except extra-virgin olive oil and organic virgin coconut oil, junk food, fast food, and nonorganic foods.

For liver-cleanse products and more information on my Thirty-Day Detox Challenge, see the Resources appendix. (Note: If you have been

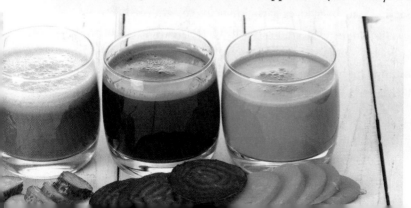

diagnosed with liver disease, consult your doctor before beginning any detox or cleansing program.)

Heavy Metals? Eat Cilantro!

Do you suffer from brain fog; insomnia; numbing, burning, or stinging sensations; pain throughout your body; memory loss; depression; muscle spasms; or chronic fatigue? If you answered yes to any of these symptoms, you may have heavy-metal deposits in your body. If you consider that every day you are bombarded by chemicals from an infinite number of sources that contain very destructive properties, it may be easy for you to see your need for a heavy-metal detox.

Heavy metals include lead, mercury, and aluminum. They contribute to the amount of neurotoxins (exogenous chemicals that destroy nerve tissue and impact hormone function) present in your body, leaving you feeling very much not like yourself.

Dr. David Williams says one of the best ways he's found to detox from neurotoxins is what he calls the "poor man's chelation therapy." He cites a study by Dr. Yoshiaki Omura with the Heart Research Foundation in New York, who "discovered a unique and easy way to remove heavy metals like mercury, lead, and aluminum."[1]

During routine antibiotic/antiviral treatment of infections Dr. Omura and his team found that after some time of showing improvement, their patients would return to them with a recurrence of the illness they had just treated. The researchers discovered that their patients had "localized deposits of mercury, lead, aluminum, or a combination, and the infectious bacterial and viral agents continued to grow and multiply in these areas."[2] With heavy metals present in the patients' bodies, the antibiotics and antivirals could not carry out their intended purpose.

During a urinalysis Dr. Omura noticed that there was a marked increase of the mercury levels in one patient's urine. The increase occurred after the patient had eaten cilantro that was added to his soup. After investigating the phenomenon a little deeper, the doctor and his team concluded that cilantro contributes to an accelerated excretion of lead, mercury, and aluminum deposits from the body. Abandoning the order of his previous protocol, Dr. Omura recommended that his patients consume cilantro—fresh or juiced—to continue the chelation of the heavy metals. They were then able to return to using antibiotics and natural antivirals to permanently heal from the infections they had.

In another study to further substantiate his cilantro remedy, Dr. Omura tested a patient who had three mercury fillings, the most common fillings American dentists have used in the past to fill cavities. Later he found "significant amounts of mercury . . . in the individual's lungs, kidneys, endocrine organs, liver, and heart," where there had been no mercury in these tissues before, and "using only cilantro, Dr. Omura was able to clear the mercury deposits in just three weeks."[3] Amazing, right?

Cilantro has demonstrated excellent results in removing heavy metals from the body. As I watched a special on Flint, Michigan's, health crisis over lead in the water, I thought about this simple remedy for the huge health problems this community has faced. How I wish I could tell every resident of Flint to start drinking cilantro juice combined with other veggie juices or to eat cilantro in soups and salads! One-fourth cup (packed) of cilantro, including stems and leaves, each day would do the trick.

But now that *you* know the remedy, you can get started with your heavy-metal detox right away. These days we are all exposed to these types of toxins all the time, and we will need a cilantro cleanse from time to time.

Just be aware that cilantro can root out heavy metals faster than your body can easily eliminate. Therefore it's important to keep them from being deposited in the colon or absorbed back into your bloodstream. To prevent this, use bentonite clay during your cilantro detox. For two weeks take 1–2 teaspoons of bentonite clay (choose the one that says "for internal use only") mixed in juice or water three times a day, between meals.

If you experience headaches, flu-like symptoms, nervousness, fever, or nausea, you should consume less cilantro to slow down the release of heavy metals but continue to take the same amount of bentonite clay. One fantastic result is greatly improved energy and a sense of well-being.

SPRING CLEANING FOR YOUR KIDNEYS

Your kidneys perform many important functions, including elimination of wastes; excretion of urine; blood-pressure regulation; and balancing your body's pH, fluid levels, and electrolytes. But they can quickly become overloaded and unable to perform their job when you choose to eat refined carbohydrates, sugar, and salt; drink too much alcohol; eat too much animal protein and fat; and consume mucus-forming foods such as dairy products. Our overreliance on prescription drugs and our exposure to pesticides, mercury, and the many other environmental toxins we encounter regularly cause damage to our kidneys as well. When our kidneys can't function at their optimal level, they become congested, and kidney stones and other kidney disorders can develop. Problems can begin when the kidneys aren't well-nourished. Being undernourished weakens them and diminishes blood flow in and out. It is important to nourish them with kidney-supporting foods such as berries, asparagus, celery, and black sesame seeds.

Notice your kidney function

The following symptoms will clue you in if your kidneys are becoming backed up and need cleansing. Pay attention if you:

+ Are unable to hold your urine (incontinence)

+ Are waking frequently throughout the night to urinate

+ Experience burning or pain during urination

+ Experience pain in your eyes

+ Feel cold in the lower half of your body

+ Have cloudy urine

+ Have foul-smelling or dark-yellow urine

+ Notice dark circles under your eyes

+ See blood in your urine

If you have even one of these symptoms, it's a good idea to cleanse and support your kidneys. They are small organs that have a mighty job to do. Too often we wait until it's crisis time before we do an intervention. Your kidneys will thank you for giving them the attention they need. And even if you have none of the symptoms of kidney congestion, it's a good idea to cleanse them once a year with cleansing juices and teas that support the kidneys.

The juices and herbs on the following list are part of your kidney cleanse week. For seven days you will include these foods in your diet.

+ The herb parsley is not often juiced and drunk alone, but together with other mild-tasting vegetable and fruit juices, such as celery, carrot, cucumber, and lemon, it serves as a good diuretic and kidney cleanser.

+ The citric acid in lemon or lime juice helps to reduce the buildup of calcium in the kidneys, which can lead to kidney stones. For a quick kidney-cleansing tonic using

lemon or lime juice, combine 2 tablespoons of freshly
squeezed lemon or lime juice with a dash of cayenne
pepper and 10–14 ounces of purified water. You will need
to drink at least one gallon of this tonic every day for three
days. To accomplish this, try to drink it throughout the
day, along with vegetable juices and herbal teas. Eat fresh
vegetables and fruits to really pump up the results.

+ Drink cranberry juice mixed with water each day for
seven days. You can use premade unsweetened cranberry
juice concentrate or unsweetened cranberry juice and add
to water according to taste, though the best option would
be to juice fresh organic cranberries. Fresh lemon juice
and a little apple juice can be added to sweeten it just a
bit. You may choose to drink only the cranberry juice
and water or add vegetable juices and eat raw vegetables
and fruits. Try to drink about 32 ounces of cranberry
water a day for that week.

+ For three days during your kidney cleanse drink water-
melon-seed tea at least once a day. Here's how to make it:
Start by pouring a pint of boiling water over 1 tablespoon
ground or chopped watermelon seeds. Allow it to steep
for five to ten minutes. After letting it cool a bit, strain it
and drink. Make this tea fresh every day.

+ For three days drink celery-seed tea once a day. To make
the tea, chop or grind fresh a tablespoon of celery seeds.
Pour a pint of boiling water over the seeds, and let the
mixture steep for five to ten minutes. After it has cooled
a bit, strain it and drink. This tea should be made fresh
each time you are ready to drink it.

+ Other teas that support the kidneys include green tea,
milk thistle tea, and nettle tea.

As you cleanse and support your kidneys and urinary tract, you will expel toxins and wastes from your kidneys. A regular kidney spring cleaning will reduce the toxic load on your kidneys and will allow them to carry on the very important work of clearing toxins from the bloodstream.

Note: Before beginning any kind of kidney cleanse, consult your health care provider, especially if you have a kidney disease. If you think you may have kidney stones or a urinary tract infection, see your doctor immediately.

THE SAUNA DETOX

We've covered the necessary spring cleaning for your intestines, liver, and kidneys due to toxic buildup, but there's another (much more fun!) way to address toxins that have built up in the body, and that's by using a sauna.

Sweating is one of the best ways to eliminate fat-soluble toxins, including perfluorocarbons (PFCs), and one of the best ways to work up a good sweat is to get in a sauna. According to some experts, saunas provide one of the few ways to detox from plastic toxins. Saunas also provide a faster way to rid your body of toxic chemicals and metals than any other detox method. By causing you to sweat profusely, saunas help to restore the skin's elimination function that often gets clogged up by an overabundance of accumulated waste.

Saunas come in two types: traditional, which includes wood-, electric-, or gas-fired, and infrared. With the traditional sauna you have to heat it up ahead of the time that you will be using it to get the temperature where you need it to be. Still, for many people, the heat that comes from the traditional sauna is often difficult to tolerate.

Because it uses ceramic heating elements, the infrared sauna does not need to be heated up before use. It is much more pleasant to use since it heats the body while the air remains cool. Sweating begins quickly with the infrared sauna. It is also known to promote better cellular elimination.

To fully benefit from either type of sauna, follow these steps:

+ Set the sauna temperature to no more than 110 degrees.

+ Before entering the sauna, drink one 16-ounce glass of fresh vegetable juice or mineralized water.

+ Do not spend more than thirty minutes at a time in the sauna, taking a ten-minute break in between sessions if you plan to return.

+ Make sure to air out the sauna whenever you use it to avoid breathing the toxic gases your body releases. A ventilation system may be built into the sauna you are using. Check the manufacturer's instructions for help with this.

+ After you exit the sauna, drink a glass of purified water.

+ Then take a warm or cool, but not hot, shower. Use a bath brush or loofa to wash off sweat and brush off dead skin cells. Brush your face and hair as well. Don't use soap, which leaves a film that clogs the pores, or traditional shampoo and hair rinse, which are loaded with chemicals. Use a natural, organic shampoo and conditioner. Avoid conventional, heavily fragranced moisturizers. Instead use organic virgin coconut oil to moisturize your skin.

+ After you shower, sit or lie down for about ten minutes.

+ To remineralize your body during your sauna detox, add extra Celtic sea salt or kelp granules to your diet.

+ Eat only organic, whole foods grown in mineral-rich soil.

+ Get plenty of rest while detoxing—at least eight hours of sleep.

+ Exercise for at least thirty minutes every day—nothing too strenuous. Light cardio such as walking is a perfect way to keep things moving.

+ Go outside, away from heavily trafficked roads, and breathe deeply the clean, fresh air.

+ Do your best to eliminate all toxic chemicals.

+ Maintain a positive attitude. As the proverb says, "A merry heart does good like medicine."

Developing a regular detoxification schedule is just like planning major seasonal house cleanings. You make a list of all the areas of your home that need extra care and a deep, thorough cleaning. You gather all your cleaning tools and supplies. You set the date and get to work. It is much the same for developing a regular fasting and detox plan for your body, mind, and spirit. Take inventory for what areas in your life or body need sprucing up. Make a list of the foods, tools, and resources you'll need. Set a time frame, and get to work. When you make the effort to invest in your overall well-being, you ensure that health, wellness, and vitality will be yours for years to come.

THE THREE-DAY FAST DETOX

Based on all the information you just learned about detoxing while fasting, you may want to give it a try. I've put together a fast-detox plan—one that you can do quickly—that will give you a sampling of what the more intense cleansing program would be like. My Thirty-Day Detox Challenge that I run throughout the year includes the Colon Cleanse, Liver-Gallbladder Cleanse with Parasite Cleanse, Kidney-Bladder Cleanse, Lung Cleanse, Skin and Blood Cleanse, and Lymphatic System Cleanse. You could start right now and give your body a little spring cleaning with this three-day fast detox.

Day 1: The Fast Colon Flush

This first day of the three-day detox targets the colon with juices and fiber that help you flush out toxins. Get rid of the waste that clogs up your "indoor plumbing." What you start today you will continue in part for the remainder of the three days because you'll want to keep your colon moving as toxins get released from your pathways of elimination.

Cleansing your intestinal tract is a great way to boost energy and vitality while improving a variety of symptoms, such as constipation, headaches, and acid reflux. Cleansing the colon is one of the most overlooked steps when it comes to losing weight, flattening the belly, and improving digestion. If your colon is congested, your digestion will be impaired, and you won't absorb nutrients efficiently. This can cause you to feel hungry a lot of the time.

You want to start with the colon cleanse because your body will pull toxins from their little hiding places. They'll be carried to the bowel for elimination. But if your bowel is congested, the toxins won't have a good escape route. That can lead to their getting absorbed back into the system, and your good efforts will be defeated. You could then experience symptoms such as headaches, rashes, fever, chills, dizziness, weakness, or fatigue. So let's get going and get that colon cleansed in short order.

Here's what you *won't* do on this day:

- Consume alcohol, coffee, nicotine, over-the-counter medications, vitamins, or supplements

- Eat meat, dairy, grains, sugar, or solid food of any kind

Here's the colon cleanse program summary:

- Drink at least 8 glasses of purified water.

- Drink vegetable juices.

- Enjoy green tea and herbal tea.

- Try a detox fiber shake.

- Have a cup of organic chicken broth, bone broth or miso broth (available at health food stores).

The Fast Colon-Flush Menu

Upon rising
Hot water with lemon
Fiber Shake (see recipe below)
Green or herbal tea (optional)

Breakfast

Colon-Flush Juice Cocktail

1 cucumber, peeled if not organic
1 handful spinach, washed
1 handful parsley, washed
1 stalk celery, washed

½ medium lemon, peeled
½ apple (green is lower in sugar)*

Bunch up the spinach and parsley, and push them through the juicer with the cucumber, celery, lemon, and apple (if using). Pour into a glass and drink as soon as possible. Serves 1.

*If you are diabetic, are hypoglycemic, or have yeast overgrowth, you may need to eliminate the apple to keep the sugar low.

Note: You will drink three to four glasses of juice on Day 1. You may repeat this recipe or choose other recipes from this book.

9:00 a.m.

Probiotic to replenish the good gut bacteria

11:00 a.m.

Fiber Shake

Lunch

Fiber Shake

2:00 p.m.

Wheatgrass Juice Pick-Me-Up

Have a 1- to 2-ounce shot of wheatgrass juice, or mix wheatgrass juice powder with water. Wheatgrass juice is very energizing. It is not recommended that you drink this after 3:00 p.m., as it can keep you awake at night.

3:00 p.m.

Fiber Shake

Dinner

Colon-Flush Juice Cocktail or a juice recipe from chapter 7. You may also have a cup of bone broth or miso broth.

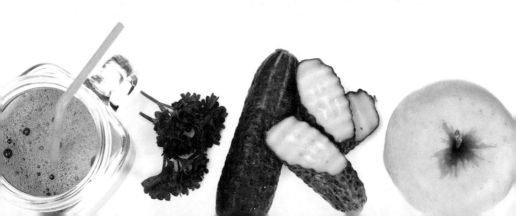

After dinner

Take a digestive stimulator; these are herbs that get the colon moving. (See the Resource appendix for more information.)

8:00 p.m.

Herbal tea and probiotic

9:00 p.m.

Fiber Shake

DIY Fiber Blend

You can either make your own fiber blend or purchase a colon-cleanse kit. (See the Resources appendix.) If you want to put together your own blend, you can purchase fiber and clay at your health-food store. To grind flaxseeds, you will need either a seed grinder or a small coffee grinder.

½ cup flax fiber or ground flaxseeds
½ cup bentonite clay (for internal use; if you get dry clay, you can mix it with the fiber blend; otherwise, you will need to mix it in water with the fiber)
2 Tbsp. ground psyllium husks or seeds
1 Tbsp. activated charcoal (optional)
2–3 Tbsp. apple or citrus pectin (optional)

Mix all these dry ingredients together and store in a cool, dry place. Makes about 1¼ cups.

Fiber Shake

To make the Fiber Shake, mix 1 to 1½ tablespoons of the DIY Fiber Blend mixture in 8 ounces of water or juice, and shake well. If you are using water, you can add flavor to the water with a teaspoon of lemon or lime juice or unsweetened cranberry juice.

Cleansing Herbs

There are many commercial colon-stimulating products that use various herbs and nutrients that keep your bowels moving. Choose a product that works well for you. The products I recommend I've tried many times and know that they work well and are not harsh for the colon. You want your bowels to move two or three times a day. You want to pull waste material off the walls of the colon and remove the impacted material.

Magnesium is an excellent mineral that helps alleviate constipation by drawing water into the intestines, causing the feces to soften. Herbs that help in colon cleansing include slippery elm bark, marshmallow root, peppermint leaf, coriander, gentian, cinnamon, rhubarb root, papaya, cayenne, spearmint, garlic, fennel, and ginger root. I don't recommend cascara sagrada or senna herbs, as they can be too irritating for the colon. However, some people are so constipated that they need a formula that includes one or both, along with more soothing herbs such as slippery elm, marshmallow root, and peppermint. Stimulating herbs can be quite beneficial during a colon cleanse but should not be used long term, as they can create dependence. (See the Resources appendix.)

Day 2: The Fast Liver Flush

The liver is your largest internal organ and the body's main organ of detoxification. It is extremely important to the body because it performs hundreds of duties each day. It processes biological functions like a busy work crew. Without a healthy, well-functioning liver you can start feeling tired, sick, run-down, and depressed. You may gain weight or not be able to lose it. Environmental pollutants, cosmetic chemicals, pesticides, medication residues, chlorine and fluoride from the water, and heavy metals all can get stored in our liver. All this junk can affect energy production. Then we begin feeling tired. The liver regulates thyroid hormone conversion and is a key organ in metabolism and weight control.

If you have a sweet tooth, listen up! Your liver will convert these calories mostly to fat and store it. You can end up with a fatty liver. It's time to flush it out and clean things up. If you're ready to brighten your skin and lose a couple of pounds, today's the day to perk up your liver.

The Fast Liver-Flush Menu

Upon rising

7:00 a.m. or upon rising
1 cup filtered water (distilled is best for detoxing)

7:15 a.m. (fifteen minutes later)

Blended Citrus Shake Liver-Gallbladder Flush

1 cup distilled or purified water
Juice of 1 lemon
Juice of 1 lime

Juice of 1 orange (optional; omit if you have diabetes, hypoglycemia, or
   yeast overgrowth)
1-inch-chunk fresh ginger root
1 clove garlic
1 Tbsp. extra-virgin, cold-pressed olive oil
2–4 ice cubes (optional; make ice cubes with filtered or distilled water)

Place all ingredients into blender and blend at high speed for about one minute
or until everything is well blended. Pour into a large glass and drink it all. This
shake will stimulate your liver and begin to flush out toxins. Serves 2.

Breakfast

Liver-Cleansing Cocktail

1 cucumber, peeled
3 carrots, scrubbed well, tops removed, ends trimmed
1 beet with stem and leaves, scrubbed well
2 ribs celery
1 handful parsley
1- to 2-inch-chunk ginger root, scrubbed or peeled if old
½ lemon, peeled

Cut produce to fit your juicer's feed tube. Juice all ingredients and stir. Pour into
a glass and drink as soon as possible. Serves 1–2.

Supplement: 1–2 capsules of the herb milk thistle or liver-cleansing
herbs.

10:00 a.m.

1 cup dandelion tea

8 oz. water with lemon (⅛–¼ lemon)

1–2 tsp. Beet Salad

Beet Salad

1 cup beet pulp

Dressing

2 Tbsp. extra virgin olive oil
1 Tbsp. fresh lemon juice
Dash of cinnamon (optional)

Whisk together and pour on beet pulp. Mix well. Serves 1.

11:30 a.m.

Ginger or echinacea herbal tea

Lunch

Beet-Berry Liver-Cleanse Cocktail

Beets are a traditional remedy for cleansing the liver.

  2 medium beets
  1 cup blueberries
  1 green apple
  2 large carrots
  1 broccoli stem
  1 lemon, peeled
  1-inch-chunk ginger
  ½ cup coconut water

Juice all ingredients. Add coconut water, stir, and enjoy. Serves 1.

1:15 p.m.
1–2 tsp. Beet Salad

3:00 p.m.

Green Drink

Juice as many greens as you like. Start with a base of cucumber, celery, and lemon. To that, add parsley, kale, spinach, sprouts, or any other greens. If juicing is not possible, mix powdered greens in water.

1–2 tsp. Beet Salad

4:30 p.m.
8 oz. water or herbal tea with lemon (⅛–¼ lemon)
1–2 tsp. Beet Salad

Dinner

Wild Greens Detox Juice

One of the best herbs to use for a liver cleanse, dandelion acts as a cleansing agent on both the liver and the kidneys. It helps to purify the blood and flush out uric acid crystals that accumulate from eating a diet

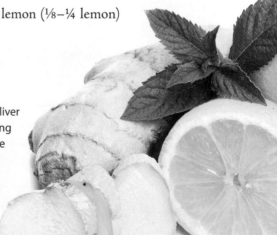

too rich in animal proteins and other acid-producing foods. It also restores the alkalinity of the blood.

> 1 cucumber, peeled if not organic
> 1 celery rib
> 1 handful wild greens, such as dandelion, nettles, plantain, lamb's
>   quarters, or sorrel
> 1 apple (green is lower in sugar)
> 1 lemon, peeled if not organic

Cut all ingredients to fit your juicer's feed tube, then juice. Stir the juice and drink as soon as possible. Serves 1.

Carrot Salad With Lemon–Olive Oil Dressing

> 1 cup carrot pulp

Dressing

> 2 Tbsp. extra-virgin olive oil
> 1 Tbsp. fresh lemon juice
> Dash of cinnamon (optional)

Whisk together and pour on carrot pulp. Mix well. Serves 1.

Vegetable salad or blended vegetable soup; you may substitute cooked artichokes, which are very liver supportive, but no dressing or dip other than olive oil and lemon juice.

Supplement: 1–2 capsules milk thistle or liver-cleansing herbs

7:15 p.m.
1–2 tsp. Beet Salad

8:30 p.m.
Chamomile or peppermint herbal tea

Day 3: The Fast Kidney-Bladder Flush

Upon rising
Drink 1 cup of herbal tea such as agrimony, marshmallow, juniper, or buchu. (These can be found at health-food stores.) These diuretic herbs will help rid the body of excess water, and they benefit the urinary tract as well.

Breakfast

Drink fresh juice such as Kidney Tonic Juice (see recipe below) or cranberry water. You also may have a green smoothie. Choose from the recipes in chapter 7. You may add a concentrated greens powder such as barley greens or wheatgrass juice powder or a blend of different green-juice powders to your juice or green smoothie.

Midmorning

Drink nettle tea.

Also, drink a glass of cranberry water. Make this by adding 1–2 tablespoons unsweetened cranberry juice to an 8- to 10-ounce glass of water. You may add a little stevia, if desired. (Do not use any artificial sweeteners, including Splenda.)

Lunch

You may have a vegetable salad, raw vegetable sticks, or lightly steamed vegetables such as broccoli or cooked artichoke, and/or you may choose from any of the juice, smoothie, or raw-soup recipes in chapter 7. For salad dressing, choose from olive oil, lemon juice, avocado, garlic, and any spices or herbs. You also may have beans, lentils, or split peas. Quinoa is excellent. Seeds and nuts are good. You may have dehydrated crackers, kale chips, zucchini chips, or dehydrated onion rings.

Midafternoon

Drink a glass of cranberry water.

Dinner

6:00 p.m.

You can repeat any vegan meals, same as lunch. See the recipes for the Daniel fast in chapter 8.

Evening

Herbal tea

Avoid eating after 7:00 p.m. to give your kidneys a chance to do their work of detoxing while you sleep.

Nettle Tea

The herb nettle is used traditionally for kidney cleansing and support; it helps eliminate uric acid. Drink 1 cup of this tea this day.

Kidney Tonic Juice

1 cucumber, peeled if not organic
1 handful parsley
1 stalk celery
¼ lemon, peeled, or a handful mint
½-inch-piece ginger root

Juice all ingredients, stir, and enjoy! Serves 1.

I hope you enjoy my quick cleanse three-day detox and want to do more. You can do the in-depth thirty-day detox, which is much more thorough and gives you a complete cleanse. See the Resources appendix for more information. And if you have questions about fasting, the next chapter should help you get some answers.

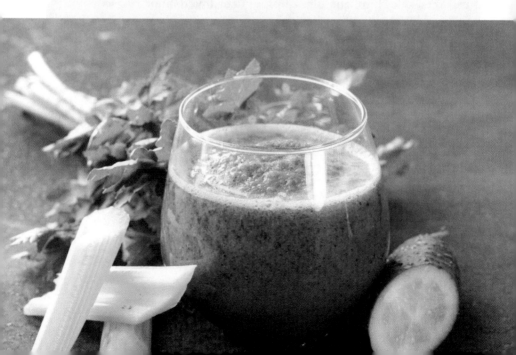

Chapter 6

FREQUENTLY ASKED QUESTIONS ABOUT FASTING

He who eats until he is sick must fast until he is well.
—ENGLISH PROVERB

MANY QUESTIONS ARISE when people are fasting. I want to address as many questions as I possibly can in this chapter so you can make your fast productive and complete on the days you choose to fast. Many people have joined my five-day juice-fast group with numerous questions. I've answered hundreds of questions on the private Facebook coaching page for that group. I think I've included here most of the ones that are frequently asked.

FAQs

How do I begin a fast? What kind of preparation do I need?

It is important to think about preparing for your fast two or three days before you actually begin it. What type of fast do you want to choose? Why do you want to fast? Write down the answers to these questions. Choose a fast that you believe is attainable for you. Write out the shopping list for the fast you've chosen.

It's also important to set your mind to complete your fast. Fasting is not easy in this country of abundance, when we're surrounded by people who would never consider fasting for one day or even one meal. You know the adage: *If you fail to plan, you plan to fail.*

You'll also want to prepare for your fast by easing into it. One of the worst things you can do is "pig out" the day before starting. It is best to eat light and healthy for at least two days—but preferably three—before you start. See chapter 2 for more details on preparing your body to fast.

115

How long should I fast?

Most people choose to fast from one to seven days for a water or juice fast and ten to forty days for the Daniel fast. Three to five days seems to be the most popular length of time for a juice or water fast.

If you have never fasted before and you are choosing a juice fast, you might want to start on the weekend, when you have more time to rest and make juice. We juice-fast together for three days at our juice-and-raw-foods retreats, which is very doable for everyone. People also find it quite helpful to juice-fast together.

Liquid fasting for longer than seven days is considered an extended fast, and you should check with your doctor to make sure you are healthy enough for an extended fast. You can, however, do a liquid fast for seven days, eat solid food for three days, and then go back on the liquid fast for seven days. If you choose the Daniel fast, an extended fast is not a problem because you are eating solid food; you simply are choosing a vegan diet.

How often should I fast?

Fasting or cleansing is most effective when done with the seasons. It is said that if you cleanse or fast at the start of each season, you probably will never get sick. I don't think there is a wrong time to fast, although you need to pick a time that is right for you. Trying to fast when there is a special occasion or holiday that calls for celebration food makes it rather difficult to stick to the fast. Always choose a time to fast that works best for you. You can make fasting part of your lifestyle and fast once a month for several days. Or you can do the intermittent fast, which is two days a week.

Can I fast during pregnancy?

Research has indicated that pregnant women can do short fasts, such as one or two days, up to the twentieth week of pregnancy, but they should not fast after that, as it could put the mother at risk of premature birth.[1] A few studies show little or no effect on newborn babies if the mother fasts. But fasting should be determined on an individual basis, depending on the health of the mother. Here's what research has shown:[2]

+ The measure of the physical condition of a newborn (known as the Apgar score) of babies born to women who fasted was no different from that of babies born to women who did not fast.

+ The birth weight of babies whose mothers fasted was only slightly lower than that of babies born to women who didn't fast.

+ Babies born to women who fasted were only slightly shorter and thinner than babies born to women who did not fast.

Can I fast if I am breastfeeding?

Research shows that short (one- to two-day) fasts have no impact on breast milk.[3] You can do short fasts while breastfeeding, but you should drink plenty of liquids. You can do the Daniel fast without any problem since it is a vegan diet.

Should I consult my doctor before fasting?

If you are taking medications or if you have health problems, it is important to consult your physician if you plan on anything more than a short fast. Everyone doing an extended water or juice fast should consult his or her doctor. Short liquid fasts and the Daniel fast should not be a problem unless you have serious health issues or are emaciated; then it is important to consult with your doctor or seek supervision for a juice fast.

Can children fast?

The age when children can begin to do short fasts is around age ten, but this depends on the health of your child. Always check with your doctor if you are unsure.

Should I exercise while fasting?

According to some experts, exercise while fasting is beneficial to your muscles. Fitness expert Ori Hofmekler says it produces "acute states of oxidative stress," which are "essential for keeping your muscle machinery tuned."[4] Hence, he goes on to say, "Exercise and fasting help counteract all the main determinants of muscle aging. But there is something else about exercise and fasting. When combined, they trigger a mechanism that recycles and rejuvenates your brain and muscle tissues."[5]

This would apply to short fasts, intermittent fasts, and the Daniel fast. If you are doing a longer period of fasting, such as three to seven days or longer, you need to consider the type of exercise you choose. A study published in 1987 found that during a three-day fast, a healthy adult could perform high-intensity exercise for thirty minutes or less. Moderate-intensity exercise could be performed for thirty to forty-five minutes.[6] If the fast restricts water, however, you should rest since exercising while dehydrated is dangerous. (I do not recommend that you ever do a fast that restricts water.)

If you fast for longer than three days, then moderate to strenuous exercise should be avoided, but you can do gentle stretching exercises and walking. At our juice-and-raw-foods retreats we offer an exercise class each day that involves stretching, walking, and specific exercises to help the body detox. The rebounder, also known as a mini trampoline, is excellent to use while fasting and detoxing. Also, the lymphasizer is very good to get the lymphatic system moving.

Are enemas or colonics beneficial when I fast?

When you fast, your body has a better chance of eliminating toxins than when you are eating regular meals. Many people find that toxins are released faster than their bodies can handle them. In such cases enemas and colonics can be very helpful in facilitating elimination of toxins. See chapter 5 for more information.

Can I take my supplements when I fast?

Usually it is not recommended that you take supplements when you fast, especially if it is a water fast or juice fast. In this case you want to give your entire digestive system a rest. Supplements require your body to work to digest them. This is why juicing is so helpful. Juice is broken down like a predigested food. Your body can absorb the nutrients easily without much work. Many supplements have fillers, and some supplements that are not high quality are almost indigestible. They create a burden for your body. However, you can use powdered or liquid supplements, as they are broken down and much easier to absorb.

Should I eat only organic produce during a fast?

When you fast, it's more important to choose organic produce than at any other time. Your body will release toxins during a fast; you don't want to add more toxins from pesticide-laced produce. The goal of fasting is to unload everything that weighs you down and burdens your body and soul.

There's a reason organic foods are more popular than ever and why sales of organics reach into the billions of dollars each year. An ever-growing number of people want to avoid their portion of the billion pounds or more of pesticides and herbicides sprayed onto crops each year.[7] More people are waking up to the fact that all these pesticides are ruining our health. It has been estimated that only 0.1 percent of applied pesticides reach the target pests; the rest is absorbed into the plants and diffused into our air, soil, and water.[8] This pesticide residue poses long-term health risks, such as cancer, Parkinson's disease, and birth defects.[9] Other immediate problems include acute intoxication, as indicated by vomiting, diarrhea, blurred vision, tremors, convulsions, and nerve damage.

We're told that pesticides and herbicides do not pose a big health risk. But consider this: when compared with the cancer rates of the general public, there is a greater incidence of cancer, particularly lymphoma, leukemia, and cancer of the brain, skin, stomach, and prostate, among crop workers and farmers and their families.[10]

Highly toxic glyphosate is sprayed on oats, wheat, barley, and other crops as a desiccant—a pesticide used to dry out crops and speed up harvesting. What's more, "Glyphosate residues are neither removed by washing nor broken down by cooking. The herbicide residue remains on food for more than a year, even if processed, dried, or frozen," says Maya Shetreat-Klein, MD, author of *The Dirt Cure: Growing Healthy Kids With Food Straight From Soil*.[11] You can't wash pesticides off. They are systemic; they're in the water of the plant, absorbed through the roots. Glyphosate is linked to cancer, Parkinson's, and Alzheimer's. This is why it is so important to purchase only organic bread, crackers, buns, rolls, oatmeal and other cereals, all other flour-based products, and beer. Yes, beer! It's made with grains.

If you can't purchase all organic fruits and vegetables, follow the Environmental Working Group's recommendations of the "Dirty Dozen" and the "Clean Fifteen." According to the organization:

> Nearly three-fourths of the 6,953 produce samples tested by the U.S. Department of Agriculture in 2014 contained pesticide residues—a surprising finding in the face of soaring consumer demand for food without synthetic chemicals.
>
> This year's update of EWG's Shopper's Guide to Pesticides in Produce reports that USDA tests found a total 146 different pesticides on thousands of fruit and vegetable samples examined in 2014. The pesticides persisted on fruits and vegetables tested by USDA—even when they were washed and, in some cases, peeled.[12]

Commercially farmed fruits and vegetables vary quite a bit in their levels of pesticide residue. Some vegetables, such as broccoli, asparagus, and onions, as well as foods with thicker peels, such as avocados, bananas, and lemons, have relatively low pesticide levels compared with other fruits and vegetables.[13]

On the other side of the coin, some vegetables and fruit don't contain large amounts of pesticides; in fact, they are quite low. Each year the Environmental Working Group releases its list of the "Dirty Dozen" fruits and vegetables, which rates fruits and vegetables from worst to best (see list to follow). Eating the least-contaminated vegetables and fruits as found on the "Clean Fifteen" list (see list to follow) will expose a person to the least pesticides. You can check it out online at www. ewg.org. When the organic vegetables or fruits that you want are not available, ask your grocer to get them. You can also look for small-operation farmers in your area and check out farmers' markets. Many small farms can't afford to use as many chemicals in farming as large commercial farms use. Another option is to order organic produce by mail, online, or through a co-op.

Avoid the "Dirty Dozen"

If you can't afford to purchase all organic produce, you can still avoid the worst pesticide-sprayed produce. The Environmental Working Group says you can cut your pesticide exposure by almost 90 percent simply by avoiding the top twelve conventionally grown fruits and vegetables that have been found to be the most contaminated. Studies have shown that eating the twelve most contaminated fruits and vegetables will, on average, expose a person to about fourteen pesticides per day. Eating the twelve least-contaminated vegetables and fruits will expose a person to fewer than two pesticides per day.[14]

The produce is listed in order of the dirtiest first. This "Dirty Dozen"—plus two more—list changes each year, so to get the current ratings, visit www.ewg.org.

1. Strawberries

2. Apples

3. Nectarines

4. Peaches

5. Celery

6. Grapes

7. Cherries

8. Spinach

9. Tomatoes

10. Sweet bell peppers

11. Cherry tomatoes

12. Cucumbers

13. Hot peppers

14. Kale/collard greens[15]

Choose the "Clean Fifteen"

These fruits and vegetables are the least contaminated by pesticides; they are ranked from highest to least contaminated:

1. Avocados

2. Sweet corn

3. Pineapples

4. Cabbage

5. Sweet peas, frozen

6. Onions

7. Asparagus

8. Mangoes

9. Papayas

10. Kiwi

11. Eggplant

12. Honeydew melon

13. Grapefruit

14. Cantaloupe

15. Cauliflower[16]

According to the Environmental Working Group, "a small amount of sweet corn, papaya and summer squash sold in the United States is produced from GE [genetically engineered] seedstock. Buy organic varieties of these crops so you can avoid GE produce."[17]

How will I get enough protein when I fast?

The only fast that may cause concern about not getting enough protein is a water fast. My juice-fast program offers amino acids but not complete protein. However, it is not something to worry about for short fasts of one week or less. You can always add protein powder and make protein shakes or green smoothies if you get especially weak.

With a juice fast many people get more nutrition than when they eat solid food. It is easier for the body to extract nutrients from liquids than to get the nutrients out of solid foods. You will consume an abundance of vitamins, enzymes, phytonutrients, minerals, and biophotons, especially if you drink around a gallon of juice each day. If you're doing the Daniel fast, you have little to worry about when it comes to protein. You can choose a variety of legumes, nuts, seeds, leafy greens, and grains. Remember, fasting helps your body heal. With a vegetable-juice fast your body will use the extra nutrients to repair, restore, and rejuvenate.

Most Americans eat more protein than they actually need. We don't need animal protein three times a day. Very few cultures eat as much protein as Americans do. Because our human body is not designed to digest and assimilate all this protein, some of it can remain undigested. Protein is acidic in its final breakdown, and therefore excess protein acidifies the body and creates an environment for illness or diseases to grow. Excess protein can also damage the kidneys.[18]

How should I break a fast?

Breaking a fast is as important as the fast itself. You can do a lot of damage to your body if you don't break your fast properly. My husband and I once did a weeklong raw-foods-and-juice fast with three days of juice fasting in the middle of the week. Afterward we went to a salad bar. We tried to be careful with our choices, but the seafood looked so delicious, we had a little of it. Within a couple of hours we both had terrible stomach cramps. It was not worth a few minutes of dining pleasure!

You have to be very careful not to overburden your digestive system after a fast. Remember, it's been resting for a while and healing. You will gain the most benefit from fasting when you break it properly. So take it slow and ease into a solid food routine if you've been on water or juice and other liquids. Even with the Daniel fast I don't recommend that you go out to dinner and order a big steak and potato or burger and fries afterward. As you make wise choices, you will find that your body responds well and continues the healing process.

One important reason to ease back into eating solid food concerns your enzymes. They have taken a vacation during your fast, or at least had a big break. Now they have to get back to work. As you introduce solid food slowly, they can step up production. Also, the mucous lining of the stomach may be more vulnerable to irritation from certain foods. It's important to introduce foods that are easy to digest. Avoid irritating substances such as coffee, fried foods, greasy foods, spicy foods, and heavy foods such as steak or hamburger. Eat small portions because overeating can do damage to your system. You can experience symptoms such as stomach cramping, nausea, and even vomiting.

If you've had an extended fast, allow four days for adjusting back to normal eating. For shorter fasts one to three days is sufficient.

Best foods for breaking a fast

Vegetable juice and fruit are good choices for breaking a water fast. To break a juice fast, use this list as a general guideline, with the first six items being best for the initial fast-breaking:

- Vegetable juices and green smoothies
- Raw fruits
- Vegetable or bone broths
- Salads with lemon juice, olive oil, and herb dressing
- Steamed vegetables and vegetable soups
- Raw vegetables and raw-food dishes
- Cooked ancient grains
- Legumes (beans, lentils, split peas)
- Nuts and seeds

Finally, you can add in:

+ Eggs

+ Meats (chicken and fish first, then red meat)

A few extra fast-breaking pointers

Listen to your body as you introduce new foods. Do you experience any adverse reactions that might signal an allergy or food intolerance? Eat slowly, and chew your food well so that you know when you are full and you can facilitate good digestion. Then stop eating, even if you have not finished all the food on your plate. Stay very in tune with your body so you can read its signals.

You can start by eating smaller meals more frequently until you return to your normal routine. The more fresh, raw foods you have, the more enzymes you'll get that will help to spare your digestive system from a lot of heavy work. Take probiotics (friendly bacteria) to aid digestion. They can be found in supplements and naturally cultured and fermented foods such as sauerkraut and miso.

How much weight will I lose on a fast?

If you do a juice fast, you may lose about a pound per day. With a water fast or the lemonade fast, you may lose a little more. With the Daniel fast, you may lose two or three pounds in a week, depending on your food choices.

What if I lose too much weight?

In cases of great toxicity the body has to eliminate a lot of toxic stuff before it can get to rebuilding the body. Some cancer patients can lose quite a bit of weight during a juice fast, but they find many benefits in the long run. However, weight loss is not always what happens. One lady attended our juice-and-raw-foods retreat after having gone through conventional cancer treatment. She had a feeding tube and was very concerned she might lose more weight at the retreat, which she said she couldn't afford to do. I told her I felt certain her body would do what it needed to do. She actually gained two pounds, while everyone else was losing weight!

People with cancer often experience what is known as *cachexia*—a wasting condition caused by the cancer. When the body is cleansed well, people who had lost a lot of weight often start putting on weight again. When there is a rapidly growing tumor, it is important to detox the body quickly. Time is of the essence. Short vegetable juice fasts can be very helpful. Fruit is not good to include, though, because cancer feeds on sugar.

What if I feel worse while I fast?

As your body detoxes, which it certainly will when you fast, you may notice some symptoms of toxins being released, such as headaches, fatigue, a spacey feeling, diarrhea, bad breath, rashes, flu-type symptoms, or some aches and pains. This is all fairly normal and a sign that toxins are being expelled from their hiding places. They usually pass through your body fairly quickly.

If you have arthritis, fibromyalgia, or any other painful condition, it may get a little worse before it gets better. This is not unusual. It's actually a good sign that your body is cleansing and healing.[19] You know that with healing, often you feel a bit worse before you get better. Always make sure you are eliminating at least twice a day. If your colon backs up, you could feel much worse. See the section on enemas and colonics in chapter 5.

What if I can't do a fast?

You will never know until you try. Often the anticipation of something is worse than actually doing it. I think you will surprise yourself at what you can do. Many people come to our retreats afraid they won't be able to make it through the five days of raw foods and juices. Everyone has come through just fine. Many people are very surprised at how well they feel when they are finished with the fast.

Will I feel weak when I fast?

Some people experience a day or two when they feel weak or tired. You may notice periods of feeling more tired because your body is cleansing and healing. Get more rest and extra sleep at these times. But overall, people actually gain energy.

I know of people who were bedridden and very sick with cancer. When I got them on an abundance of fresh vegetable juices, they were greatly helped. I worked with one man who was up and riding around his property on his golf cart within a few days of being on the juices and raw foods. So far I've not encountered anyone who couldn't do a juice fast. One lady who came to our retreat in a wheelchair and who had been bedridden before coming was walking by the fourth day.

Remember, when you fast with juices, the nutrients are already broken down and your body doesn't have to work very hard to get nutrition. With the Daniel fast the body has to work a little harder but not as hard as it does on a regular meat-centered diet.

Will my blood sugar get too low?

If you juice vegetables, minimize the higher-sugar veggies such as carrots and beets, and don't use fruit except for lemon or lime and low-sugar fruits such as berries and green apple, you should be just fine. I'm one who is prone to low blood sugar, so this is how I juice. I choose lots of green veggies, including cucumber, celery, leafy greens such as chard or kale, and parsley. I include ginger and lemon. If I can find turmeric root, I juice some of that. And I often include a few carrots.

I also have a partly blended juice cocktail I make with frozen tomato chunks. I juice carrots and lemon and pour that in my blender over the frozen tomato chunks. I add at least ¼ cup of cilantro with a dash of sea salt and a pinch of cayenne pepper. Then I blend and enjoy. This is very grounding for me.

A pinch of sea salt definitely helps if you start feeling weak or dizzy. Often tiredness can be interpreted as low blood sugar, but it's actually part of the cleansing reaction. I've never had my blood sugar get too low when I watch the produce I choose and juice only vegetables with lemon or lime. The key is not to get too much sugar if you are prone to low blood sugar. The one caution is if you have diabetes. (See the answer to the next question.)

Can I fast if I have diabetes or hypoglycemia?

If you have diabetes and want to do a juice fast, use no fruit except for lemon or lime juice and cranberries, tomatoes, and avocado (which won't juice, but you can make green smoothies with it). Juice lots of green vegetables, and include green beans. You should test your blood sugar at least three times a day. Your blood sugar can drop very quickly on a juice fast, so your regular dose of insulin can cause it to drop too low. You want to be very aware of this and adjust your insulin or other blood-sugar-lowering medication. You may also experience peaks in blood sugar. If your blood sugar drops too low, then a little orange juice can be helpful to bring it back up. If you feel weak or dizzy, you could eat a little avocado and/or add a pinch of sea salt. Also, minimize carrots and beets; they are higher-sugar vegetables.

Most diabetics can do short veggie-juice fasts. You should have no problem doing the Daniel fast. I do not recommend a water fast or the lemonade fast for anyone with sugar-metabolism problems.

Can I drink smoothies on my juice fast?

You may combine green smoothies with juice for a juice-and-smoothie fast. This works well for many people who get weak or faint when they try to juice fast as well as people who have demanding jobs. You'll still gain a lot of benefit from this type of fast. See chapter 7 for menus and recipes.

Chapter 7

THE QUICK AND EASY JUICE-FAST MENU AND RECIPES

Through abstinence, what is tired and
weak and sick becomes strong.
—HYMN SUNG BY MONKS DURING LENT

YOU MAY CHOOSE to fast from one to seven days. Actually you can juice-fast for longer periods of time, but you may want to check with your doctor for extended periods of fasting. I've had people who joined my Thirty-Day Detox Challenge decide on a juice fast for all thirty days with great results. Listen to your body's wisdom. This is an opportunity to give your body a break from digesting all the food you normally eat. When the body isn't focused on digesting solid food, it can focus on healing and repair. Juice fasting rejuvenates your body right down to your cells. That's why many people notice that wrinkles disappear and they look younger and more vibrant. Talk about encouraging! This is your opportunity to restore your body as well as your soul and spirit.

TIPS FOR EFFECTIVE JUICE FASTING

Back when I first started juice fasting, I was so determined to get well, I just went for it. I didn't care how I felt. I was committed to fasting to get well. Then I kept on fasting year after year to stay healthy. I learned that:

+ I could do this, even though I wasn't sure I could when I started.

+ When it got tough through the fast, I found out I could make it, one hour, one day at a time.

+ I looked at fasting as a new discovery. I was very curious
   about what I would experience physically.

Now it's your turn. You're about to experience what juice fasting has
in store for you.

Need a Protein Powder Boost? Choose Your Protein Wisely

If you are doing a juice fast or juice-and-smoothie fast, you may need some protein to keep going on busy workdays. Whatever you choose, look at the sweeteners and fillers. I recommend powders sweetened with stevia. I don't recommend soy protein, due to the fact that soy is a goitrogen, meaning an iodine blocker. This can adversely affect your thyroid. It's also the largest GMO crop in the United States. Here's what I do recommend:

WHEY PROTEIN

If you aren't dairy sensitive, whey protein is considered the most complete protein. It can enter your bloodstream faster than other protein powders. It's also known to be good for helping to build muscle. Choose an organic powder made from milk of grass-fed cows.

PEA PROTEIN

This protein powder is made from yellow peas and has a light, fluffy texture. It is known to be the most digestive of the plant protein powders. This is a good alternative for anyone who doesn't choose to do dairy. Being low in two amino acids, it's not a complete protein, but if you mix it with another plant protein such as hemp or rice, then it is complete.

HEMP PROTEIN

Low in amino acids, just 10 to 15 grams per scoop, hemp protein is not the best for building muscle. But it's a good source of fiber and omega-3 fatty acids. Combine it with pea or rice protein for a complete protein.

RICE PROTEIN

Rice protein has a more distinct taste than other protein powders—not as smooth and a bit chalky. Mix it with pea protein, and you have a complete protein as well as improved texture and flavor.

THE BASIC JUICE-FAST MENU

This is your basic juice-fast menu plan. You will want to drink at least three large (12-ounce) glasses of juice per day, but you'll do better with drinking two quarts to a gallon of juice, depending on your size. You can try a variety of juice recipes or find your favorite few and stick with them. Whatever you decide is great. If you find that you need encouragement and support, you can join my juice-fast online group. I have one going each month that includes private Facebook coaching and a weekly teleconference call during which you can ask questions.

Start your day

Drink 8 ounces of purified water first thing in the morning. It will flush your liver.

Next up

Drink a cup of hot water and lemon with a dash of cayenne. This will get your liver moving in the morning. Also, lemon is thought to cleanse the digestive tract.

Breakfast

Pick your juice recipe from the juice recipe section in this chapter.

Midmorning pick-me-up

Drink wheatgrass juice or wheatgrass juice powder mixed in purified water—wheatgrass juice is an excellent pick-me-up for the midmorning—or you can have coconut water or herbal tea.

Lunch

Pick your juice recipe.

Midafternoon rejuvenator

Drink wheatgrass juice or wheatgrass juice powder mixed in purified water, or you can have coconut water or herbal tea.

Dinner

Pick your juice recipe.

Evening calming tea

Drink a cup of chamomile or chamomile lavender tea (or any other favorite herbal tea).

Don't Forget to Drink Water

Make sure you drink at least eight glasses of purified water each day. This is especially important when you are fasting, to flush away toxins. See chapter 3 for more information on the importance of water when fasting.

THE WEEKEND FAST FLUSH

Renew, revive, and refresh your body in just a weekend! You may want to try this simple three-day juice fast to lose weight or to look more vibrant for a special event. These juices really help melt the pounds away, so give it a try.

Each day of this fast I emphasize a different color theme of juices. I call it the weekend fast, but you can do it anytime. However, if you have a busy workweek, you might want to start the fast on Friday and end it Sunday evening. That way you'll have the weekend for making juice and giving yourself extra rest at the same time.

I think you'll find this fast is a lot of fun. You can switch recipes around as you like. I gave you a number of fun recipes to help you get started, but please know you aren't locked into any ingredient or recipe. People often ask me if they can substitute one ingredient for another. You can always make substitutions! (If you are diabetic, are hypoglycemic, or have yeast overgrowth or cancer, though, you should eliminate the apple to keep your sugar low.) You don't even need to stick with my color theme. Make this three-day fast work for you. If you find a couple of recipes you really like, you can repeat them over and over. Enjoy your three-day fasting journey!

Day 1: Relish the red

When you think of red produce, the nutrient that stands out is lycopene, which is a carotenoid that is a powerful antioxidant associated with reduced cancer risk, especially prostate cancer. It is also associated with reduced risk of heart attacks. Many red fruits and vegetables are also rich in vitamin C and folate, along with flavonoids, which have been shown to reduce inflammation. Cranberries are a good source of tannins, which prevent bacteria from sticking to cells; hence they are important in fighting infections and are the reason cranberry juice is a standard treatment for bladder infections. The color red (and purple) is associated with the adrenal glands, the lymphatic system, and the kidneys.

Upon rising

Drink hot water with lemon or an herbal tea.

Breakfast

Red Sunrise

"Drinking beet juice may help to lower blood pressure in a matter of hours. One study found that drinking one glass of beet juice lowered systolic blood pressure by an average of 4–5 points."[1]

1 green apple
½ small beet with leaves
1 cucumber, peeled if not organic

Cut produce to fit your juicer's feed tube. Juice ingredients and stir. Serves 1.

Morning break

Drink hibiscus tea. (Hibiscus has anti-inflammatory properties.)

Lunch

Rosy Glow

All red, orange, and green vegetables and fruit are rich in carotenoids. Studies show that carotenoids give your skin an attractive rosy glow, even more appealing than being out in the sun.

4–5 medium carrots, tops removed
1 red apple
1 medium cucumber, peeled if not organic
1 small beet, with or without a few tops
2 ribs celery
1-inch-chunk ginger root

Juice all ingredients, stir, and enjoy! Serves 1–2.

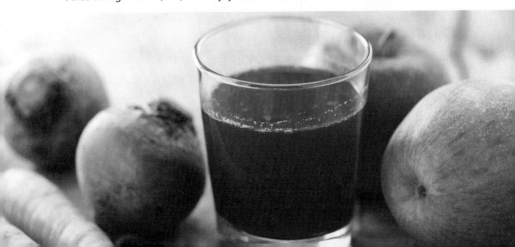

3:00 p.m. pick-me-up

Revitalizing Tomato-Coconut Juice

Coconut water is rich in electrolytes, which revitalize the body. If you can't make this juice recipe, drink a glass of coconut water.

> 1 cup carrot juice (about 6 medium carrots)
> Juice of 1 lemon
> 1 tomato, cut into chunks and frozen
> 1 large handful cilantro
> ½ cup coconut water

Pour carrot and lemon juice into a blender. Add the frozen tomato chunks and cilantro. Blend until the tomato chunks are completely processed. Stir in the coconut water. Pour into glasses, and be revitalized. Serves 2.

Dinner

Red Cabbage-Jicama-Carrot-Lime Cocktail

"The rich red color of red cabbage reflects its concentration of anthocyanin polyphenols, which contribute to red cabbage containing significantly more protective phytonutrients than green cabbage."[2]

> 1 handful flat-leaf parsley leaves
> 1 green lettuce leaf
> 3–4 carrots, scrubbed well, tops removed, ends trimmed
> 2-inch by 4- to 5-inch-chunk jicama, scrubbed well or peeled
> ¼ small red cabbage 1 lime, peeled if not organic

Cut produce to fit your juicer's feed tube. Wrap parsley in lettuce leaf and push through juicer slowly. Juice remaining ingredients. Pour into a glass and stir. Serves 1.

Day 2: Gravitate toward green

Chlorophyll is the plant pigment that gives vegetables and fruit their green color. Chlorophyll is a blood purifier. Green foods are rich in isothiocyanates, which generate enzymes in the liver that assist the body in removing carcinogenic compounds. Cruciferous veggies such as broccoli, cabbage, and brussels sprouts contain the phytonutrients indoles and isothiocyanates, which have anticancer properties. And sulforaphane, which is a phytochemical in cruciferous vegetables, has been shown to detoxify cancer-causing chemicals before they can damage your body.[3]

Drink hot water with lemon or green tea.

Green Power Morning

"Abundant flavonoids in spinach act as antioxidants to keep cholesterol from oxidizing and protect your body from free radicals, particularly in the colon."[4]

    3 carrots, scrubbed well, tops removed, ends trimmed
    2 ribs celery with leaves
    1 handful spinach
    1 cucumber, peeled if not organic
    ½ green apple

Cut produce to fit your juicer's feed tube. Juice all ingredients and stir. Pour into a glass and drink as soon as possible. Serves 1.

Drink green tea, hot or iced.

Tomato Florentine With a Twist

"*Orientin* and *vicenin* are two water-soluble flavonoids that have been of particular interest in basil, and in studies on human white blood cells; these components of basil protect cell structures as well as chromosomes from radiation and oxygen-based damage."[5]

    2 vine-ripened tomatoes
    4–5 sprigs basil
    1 large handful spinach
    1 lemon or lime, peeled if not organic

Juice one tomato. Wrap the basil in several spinach leaves. Turn off the machine and add the spinach and basil. Turn the machine back on and gently tap to juice them. Juice the remaining tomato and lemon. Stir juice, pour into a glass, and drink as soon as possible. Serves 1.

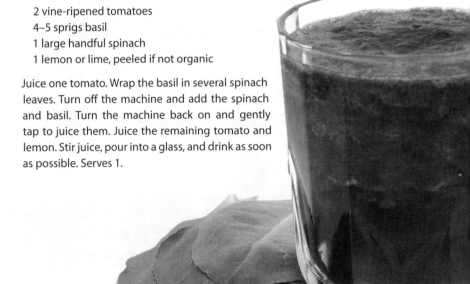

3:00 p.m. pick-me-up

Dandelion-Coconut Water

Dandelion is excellent to help detoxify the liver; however, the greens are quite bitter. The coconut water and apple do help the taste buds.

1 bunch dandelion greens
1 lime, peeled if not organic
½ green apple
1 cup coconut water

Juice the dandelion greens, lime, and apple. Stir in coconut water, and serve immediately. Serves 1.

Dinner

Refreshing Mint Cooler

Mint is a proven effective remedy for nausea.

1 fennel bulb and fronds
1 cucumber, peeled if not organic
1 green apple, such as Granny Smith or pippin
1 handful mint

Cut produce to fit your juicer's feed tube. Juice ingredients and stir. Pour into a glass over ice, and drink as soon as possible. Serves 1–2.

Day 3: Opt-in for orange

Orange and yellow foods are particularly rich in carotenes. These phytonutrients include beta-cryptoxanthin, beta-carotene, and alpha-carotene, which are converted in the body to vitamin A as needed. These nutrients are important for vision, the immune system, and the skin. These foods are rich in vitamin C and are also known to help prevent cancer.

Upon rising

Drink hot water with lemon or green tea.

Breakfast

Happy-Mood Morning

Fennel juice has been used as a traditional tonic to help the body release endorphins, the "feel-good" peptides, from the brain into the bloodstream. Endorphins help to diminish anxiety and fear, and they generate a mood of euphoria.

½ apple (green is lower in sugar)
4–5 carrots, well scrubbed, tops removed, ends trimmed
3 fennel stalks with leaves and flowers
½ cucumber, peeled if not organic
1 handful spinach
1-inch-chunk ginger root

Cut produce to fit your juicer's feed tube. Juice apple first, and follow with other ingredients. Stir and pour into a glass; drink as soon as possible. Serves 1–2.

Morning break

Drink ginger tea. (Note: Ginger is an anti-inflammatory.)

Lunch

Carrot and Spice

Regular consumption of carrots has been shown to lower cholesterol.

2–3 carrots, scrubbed well, tops removed, ends trimmed
1 handful spinach
1 cucumber, peeled if not organic
½ lemon, peeled if not organic
½ apple (green has less sugar)
1-inch-chunk ginger root
½ tsp. cinnamon
Dash cayenne pepper

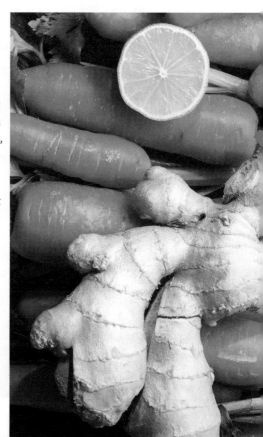

Cut produce to fit your juicer's feed tube. Juice all ingredients. Add spices and stir. Pour the juice into two glasses, and drink as soon as possible. Serves 2.

3:00 p.m. pick-me-up

Enjoy a glass of lemon-mint water or coconut water.

Dinner

The Ginger Hopper With a Twist

"Research in Italy found that those who ate more carrots had ⅓ as high a risk of heart attack as compared with those who ate less carrots."[6]

> 5 medium carrots, scrubbed well, tops removed, ends trimmed
> 1 green apple
> 1-inch-chunk fresh ginger root, peeled
> ½ lemon, peeled if not organic

Cut produce to fit your juicer's feed tube. Juice ingredients and stir. Pour into a glass, and drink as soon as possible. Serves 1.

JUICE RECIPES

I have put together a collection of recipes that have lots of different punchy flavors to keep your taste buds from frowning, plus a sprinkle of zip to change things up a bit. I also have included some basic recipes. If you rotate the recipes, you'll keep from getting bored. But if you do get bored, get my book *The Juice Lady's Big Book of Juices and Green Smoothies*, which has more than four hundred recipes in it.

Get Your Ginger Greens On

One study found that people who took 2 grams of ginger a day saw improvement in muscle pain.[7]

> 1 green apple
> ½ large fennel with fronds
> 1-inch-piece ginger root
> 1 large broccoli stem
> 1 rib celery
> 3 leaves kale
> ½ cucumber, peeled if not organic

Cut produce to fit your juicer. Start by juicing the apple and finish with the cucumber. Drink as soon as possible. Serves 1.

Immune Booster Shot

Feeling a bit down or under the weather? Give your immune system a reboot with these anti-inflammatory foods.

> 1-inch-chunk ginger
> 1-inch-chunk turmeric

Juice of 1 lemon

1 Tbsp. raw honey (or several drops liquid stevia)

Juice ginger and turmeric. Mix with juice of lemon and sweetener. Serve immediately. Serves 1.

Anti-Inflammatory Power Cocktail

In numerous studies, curcumin, which is responsible for turmeric's yellow-orange pigment, has shown "anti-inflammatory effects…to be comparable to the potent drugs hydrocortisone and phenylbutazone as well as over-the-counter anti-inflammatory agents such as Motrin."[8]

1 cucumber, peeled if not organic

2 carrots, green tops removed

1 broccoli stem

½ green apple

1-inch-piece fresh turmeric root

1-inch-piece ginger root

Juice all ingredients and give it a stir! Enjoy. Serves 1–2.

Fat Flush Ambrosia

According to research, grapefruit contains a fat-burning phytochemical that works to balance insulin levels. That means you'll burn more fat than you'll store. Grapefruit has also been shown to lower the bad (LDL) cholesterol.

1 grapefruit, peeled*

1 orange, peeled

1 small handful mint

3 leaves romaine lettuce

Juice all ingredients and give it a stir! Serves 1.

*Note: Always peel grapefruit (and oranges), as they contain volatile oils that can make you sick.

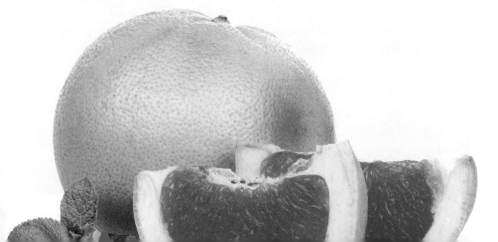

Metabolism Booster Juice

Celery and hot peppers are considered thermogenic foods, which means they boost your metabolism.

4 ribs celery with leaves
1 green apple
1 cucumber, peeled if not organic
Dash cayenne pepper or hot sauce

Juice all ingredients and give it a stir! Serves 1.

Fire and Ice

Want to kick your metabolism into high gear? Add more chili peppers. They contain capsaicin, which is a chemical compound that can rev up your metabolism.

2 green apples
6 kale leaves
1 cucumber, peeled if not organic
¼ jalapeño

Juice all ingredients, pour over ice, stir, and enjoy! Serves 1–2.

Don't Get Caught With Your Adrenals Down

Adrenal fatigue can ruin your life. If you have a serious case of stressed-out adrenal glands, you may have difficulty getting out of bed in the morning. In fact, you may want to sleep a good portion of your day.

With diminished adrenal function, the other organs, glands, and systems of your body are affected as well. You will experience changes in carbohydrate, protein, and fat metabolism, along with fluid and electrolyte balance and even sex drive. You can be affected right down to your cells.

The body will work hard to make up for tired adrenal glands, but your body will pay a price. Find out if you have adrenal fatigue. Take my quiz online at http://www.juiceladycherie.com/Juice/adrenal-fatigue-quiz/. If it does appear your adrenals are low, get my book *The Juice Lady's Remedies for Stress and Adrenal Fatigue*.

Adrenal Booster Cocktail

Hot peppers and parsley are rich in vitamin C; celery is a great source of natural sodium. Both nutrients are beneficial for the adrenal glands.

4 carrots, scrubbed well, green tops removed, ends trimmed
2 tomatoes

2 ribs celery
1 handful parsley
Dash hot sauce (made from hot peppers)
Dash celery salt

Cut produce to fit your juicer's feed tube. Juice ingredients and stir. Pour into a glass, and drink as soon as possible. Serves 2.

Liver Detox Juice Cocktail

One of the unique cleansing properties of arugula is that it counteracts the destructive effects of heavy metals, particularly in the liver. A member of the cruciferous vegetable family, it is rich in detoxifying antioxidants.

1 cucumber, peeled if not organic
1 handful arugula
½ cup blueberries
½ green apple
¼ cup mint
Juice of 1 lime
1-inch-chunk ginger root

Cut produce to fit your juicer's feed tube. Juice and stir. Enjoy! Serves 1.

Refreshing Rejuvenator

Cucumbers are known to be refreshing and hydrating. In fact, Middle Eastern caravans would take cucumbers with them while crossing desert terrain because they were thirst quenching and refreshing.

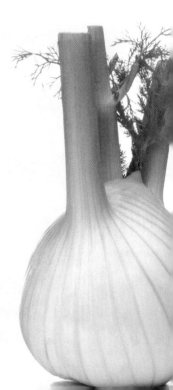

1 lime, peeled if not organic
2 green apples
1 cucumber, peeled if not organic
1 oz. wheatgrass juice or 1 serving wheatgrass juice
    powder

Juice the lime, apples, and cucumber. Stir in the wheatgrass, and enjoy! Serves 1.

The Feel Good Cocktail

Fennel is a traditional remedy for elevating the mood.

½ fennel bulb with fronds and flowers
1 cucumber
½ lemon

Juice all ingredients, stir, and enjoy! Serves 1.

Love That Garlic!

"When it comes to weight loss, garlic appears to be a miracle food. A team of doctors at Israel's Tel Hashomer Hospital conducted a test on rats to find out how garlic can prevent diabetes and heart attacks, and they found an interesting side effect—none of the rats given allicin (a compound in garlic) gained weight."[9]

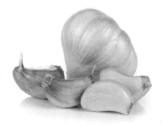

"Garlic is a known appetite suppressant. The strong odor of garlic stimulates the satiety center in the brain, thereby reducing feelings of hunger. It also increases the brain's sensitivity to leptin, a hormone produced by fat cells that controls appetite. Further, garlic stimulates the nervous system to release hormones that speed up metabolic rate such as adrenaline. This means a greater ability to burn calories. More calories burned means less weight gained—a terrific correlation."[10]

Garlic Love Weight Loss Cocktail

1–3 cloves garlic
1-inch-piece fresh ginger
6–7 carrots, tops removed
½ green apple

Juice all ingredients and stir. Enjoy! Serves 1.

Blood-Sugar-Balancing Cocktail

Green beans are helpful for the pancreas and the stability of blood sugar.

2 romaine lettuce leaves
1 cucumber, peeled if not organic
1 celery rib
8–10 string beans
½ lemon, peeled
¼ tsp. cinnamon
1 carrot

Bunch up romaine lettuce leaves. Cut produce to fit your juicer's feed tube. Tuck the romaine lettuce in the feed tube, and push it through with the cucumber. Juice remaining ingredients, finishing with the carrot. Pour into a glass and enjoy! Serves 1.

Curb-Your-Carb-Cravings Juice

Jerusalem artichoke juice combined with carrot and beet is a traditional remedy for satisfying cravings for sweets and junk food. The key is to sip it slowly when you get a craving for high-fat or high-carb foods.

1 Jerusalem artichoke, scrubbed well
3–4 carrots, scrubbed well, tops removed, ends trimmed
½ small beet, scrubbed well
½ cucumber, peeled if not organic
½ lemon, peeled if not organic

Cut produce to fit your juicer's feed tube. Juice ingredients and stir. Pour into a glass, and drink as soon as possible. Serves 1.

Cilantro Heavy-Metal-Detox Cocktail

Cilantro has been shown in studies to help the body detox heavy metals such as mercury, lead, and aluminum.

2 tomatoes, cut in chunks
1 cup fresh carrot juice (about 5–7 carrots)
1 lemon, juiced, peeled (if putting it through a juice machine)
¼ cup cilantro, rinsed and chopped
¼ tsp. Celtic sea salt
¼ tsp. ground cumin
¼ small jalapeño, chopped (more if you like it hot)
3 radishes

Place the tomato chunks in a freezer bag and freeze until solid. This is optional. (Or you can use fresh tomatoes placed in the blender.) Pour the carrot and lemon juices into a blender, and add the frozen tomato chunks, cilantro, salt, cumin, jalapeño, and radishes. Blend on high speed until smooth but slushy; serve immediately. Serves 2.

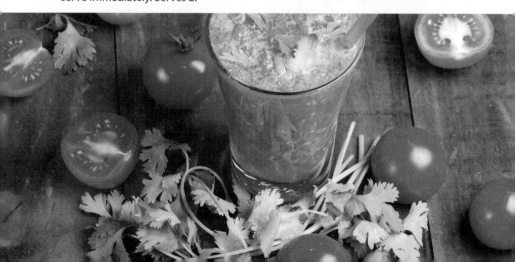

Skinny-Sip Sparkling Lemonade

With less than 10 calories, this is an ideal low-calorie, vitamin C–rich thirst quencher.

½ lemon, washed or peeled if not organic
1 cup unsweetened mineral water
2 or 3 drops liquid stevia (try SweetLeaf Vanilla Crème)

Juice the lemon, and pour the juice into a glass. Add the mineral water, and stir to combine. Sweeten with stevia to taste. Add ice as desired, or serve chilled. Serves 1.

Cholesterol-Lowering Juice Cocktail

A 2008 study showed that ginger root contributed to a significant reduction in triglycerides, cholesterol, low-density lipoprotein (LDL), and very-low-density lipoprotein (VLDL).[11]

1-inch-chunk ginger root
1 cucumber, peeled if not organic
4 carrots
1 lemon
1 green apple

Juice all ingredients, stir, and enjoy! Serves 1.

Wild Greens Detox Juice

1 cucumber, peeled if not organic
1 celery rib
1 handful wild greens (such as dandelion, nettles, plantain, lamb's
    quarters, or sorrel)
1 apple (green is lower in sugar)
1 lemon, peeled if not organic

Cut all ingredients to fit your juicer's feed tube, then juice. Stir the juice, and drink as soon as possible. Serves 1. (This recipe is included in The Fast Liver Flush described in chapter 5.)

Kidney-Cleansing Cocktail

Asparagus is a natural diuretic and great for cleansing and nourishing the kidneys.

    2 carrots, green tops removed
    1 cucumber, peeled if not organic
    8 asparagus stems
    Handful wild greens (such as dandelion greens or stinging nettles, or
        substitute arugula)
    1 lemon, peeled if not organic

Cut produce to fit your juicer's feed tube. Juice all ingredients and stir. Pour into a glass and enjoy! Serves 1–2.

Prickly Pink

This cactus fruit sports a pretty fuchsia pink color and tastes a bit like melon or bubblegum. Prickly pears are rich in potassium and magnesium—important minerals in regulating the heart.

    Prickly pears (they are small; it takes quite a few to make a glass of juice,
        and the number varies)
    Juice of 1 lime

Use gloves when removing spines and hard skin from the prickly pears. Most juicers can handle the seeds. Juice ingredients, stir, and enjoy! Serves 1.

Spicy Veggie

Curry powder is a popular spice that has been shown to prevent cancer.

    1 tomato
    1 cucumber, peeled if not organic
    ½ lemon, peeled if not organic
    2 chard leaves
    1-inch-chunk ginger
    ½ tsp. curry

Juice tomato, cucumber, lemon, chard leaves, and ginger. Stir in curry. Enjoy! Serves 1–2.

Ginger Limeade

In a 2015 study ginger was found to lower fasting blood-sugar levels as well as inflammation.[12]

    2 apples
    ½ cucumber, peeled if not organic
    1 lime, peeled if not organic
    1-inch-chunk ginger root

Juice all ingredients, stir, and enjoy! Serves 1.

Green Muscle Mender

Are you strength training? Spinach helps your muscles recover.

    1 large handful spinach
    1 green apple
    1 cucumber
    1-inch-chunk ginger root
    2-inch-piece fresh turmeric root (optional)

Juice all ingredients, stir, and enjoy! Serves 1.

Rosy Glow

Studies show that carotenoids give your skin an attractive, rosy glow—even more appealing than being out in the sun.

    4–5 medium carrots, tops removed
    1 red apple
    1 medium cucumber
    1 small beet, with or without a couple of tops
    2 ribs celery
    1-inch-chunk ginger root

Juice all ingredients, stir, and enjoy! Serves 1–2.

Carrot Cake

To get the full benefit of carotenoids from carrots, it's best to combine them with fat. Adding coconut milk is a perfect combination and so delicious, I call it carrot cake.

    5–9 large carrots, tops removed
    1 apple
    ½ cup coconut milk
    ½ tsp. cinnamon
    ¼ tsp. nutmeg

Juice carrots and apple, and pour the juice in a glass. Stir in the coconut milk, cinnamon, and nutmeg. (Make sure you use coconut milk and not coconut water to give the juice a creamy texture.) Serves 1.

Apple Pie à la Mode

"A 2003 study in the journal *Diabetes Care* showed that cinnamon may cause muscle and liver cells to respond more readily to insulin, thereby improving weight loss. Better response to insulin means better blood sugar balance and, therefore, less insulin released into your body."[13]

2 apples
1-inch-chunk ginger root
1 cup coconut milk
½ tsp. cinnamon
¼ tsp. nutmeg

Juice apples and ginger. Stir in coconut milk and spices, and enjoy! Serves 1.

Beet-Berry Liver-Cleanse Juice

Beets have been used as a natural remedy for liver cleansing.

2 medium beets
1 cup blueberries
1 green apple
1 large carrot
1 broccoli stem
1 lemon, peeled
1-inch-chunk ginger
½ cup coconut water

Juice all ingredients, except coconut water. Add coconut water, stir, and enjoy! Serves 1–2.

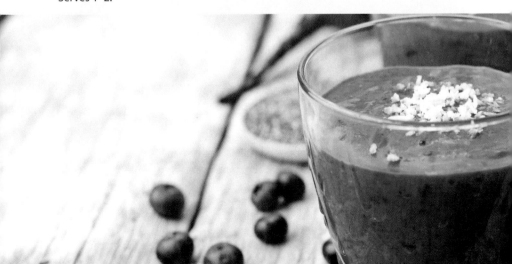

Pink Ginger Lady

One study with 261 patients found that 63 percent of the participants who had osteoarthritis of the knee experienced improvement in pain by including ginger extract in their diet.[14]

> 2 green apples
> ½ cucumber
> ¼ beet
> 1-inch-chunk ginger root

Juice all ingredients, stir, and enjoy! Serves 1.

HEALING TEAS

Lemon balm is a tea for lifting your spirits. You might need that when you're fasting! It's good for the cloudy-day blahs, which you can get even when the sun is shining.

Bilberry (huckleberry) is great for helping to balance blood sugar.

Ginger works to reduce inflammation and settle the stomach.

Sage has many medicinal uses. One of them is to help your body utilize insulin. Studies show that sage can boost insulin activity in diabetics.

SMOOTHIE AND RAW-SOUP RECIPES

You may want to add smoothies and raw soups to your juice-fast menu plan if you find you need a little extra protein and calories while you fast. You may follow the juice-and-smoothie-fast plan that follows. Integrate these recipes into your menu plan as needed.

Smoothie recipes

Strawberry-Kale Smoothie Supreme

> ½ ripe avocado
> 1 medium-ripe banana, fresh or frozen
> 1 cup fresh or frozen strawberries
> 2 large handfuls baby spinach
> 1 large kale leaf, chopped
> 1 small handful parsley, chopped
> 1½ cups unsweetened plant milk or coconut water
> 1 Tbsp. hemp or flaxseeds

Toppers:

    Blackberries
    Blueberries
    Goji berries
    Sunflower seeds
    Chia seeds
    Sesame seeds

Blend all ingredients. Serves 2.

Shamrock Green Detox Shake

The chlorophyll in dark leafy greens such as spinach helps to cleanse your body of toxins including pesticides, heavy metals, preservatives, and smog. Add some broccoli sprouts, and you'll have a wallop of antioxidant nutrients known to stimulate detoxification enzymes that support the pathways of elimination.

    ½ cup almond milk
    1 cup baby spinach
    Small handful broccoli sprouts (optional)
    ½ cucumber, peeled if not organic
    1 frozen banana
    1 Tbsp. shelled hemp seeds (some refer to them as hemp hearts)
    1 tsp. pure vanilla extract
    Handful ice cubes

Blend all ingredients until smooth. Pour into a glass, and serve immediately. Garnish with a dash of cinnamon. Serves 1–2.

Creamy Green Smoothie Bowl

Spinach, kale, and avocado bring plenty of green goodness, while coconut milk provides good fat, and hemp milk and hemp seeds add both extra protein and omega-3s for a thick, creamy treat anyone can enjoy. We serve this smoothie for the first breakfast at our retreats.

    1 cucumber, cut into chunks, peeled if not organic
    1 cup raw spinach
    1 avocado, peeled, seeded, and cut in quarters
    ½ pear
    ½ cup coconut milk or hemp milk
    Juice of 1 lime
    Chopped almonds or hemp seeds for topping (optional)

Combine all ingredients in a blender and process until creamy. Pour in a bowl and eat with a spoon. This is great served with chopped almonds on top. Serves 2.

Raw soups

Creamy Basil-Cumin-Carrot Soup

"In one study, cumin was shown to protect laboratory animals from developing stomach or liver tumors. This cancer-protective effect may be due to cumin's potent free radical scavenging abilities as well as the ability it has shown to enhance the liver's detoxification enzymes."[15]

3 cups fresh carrot juice
1 large avocado, peeled, seeded, and cut in quarters
1 green onion, chopped
Fresh basil, chopped
Juice of ½ lemon
½ tsp. cumin

Make carrot juice. Place carrot juice and avocado in food processor or blender with onion and basil. Blend until smooth. Add lemon juice and cumin, and blend. Garnish with sprouts or grated vegetables such as zucchini, cucumber, red pepper, carrots, or beets. Serves 2.

Note: This soup makes a great salad dressing also.

Creamy Carrot-Ginger-Lime Soup

Want to improve your vision? Carrots, replete with carotenoids, are excellent for the eyes. We serve this cold soup at our retreat. It's one of the favorites of the week.

3 cups carrot juice
1 avocado, peeled, seeded, and cut in quarters
¼ cup lime juice
1 Tbsp. coconut nectar (optional)

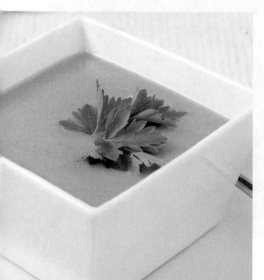

1 Tbsp. ginger, peeled and minced
¼ tsp. sea salt
¼ small shallot, minced

Make carrot juice. Place carrot juice and avocado in blender or food processor with remaining ingredients. Blend until smooth and serve. Serves 2.

Creamy Zucchini Soup With Chopped Almonds

In numerous studies zucchini was found to contain properties that effectively treat and reduce symptoms of BPH (benign prostatic hypertrophy), which is an enlarged prostate.[16]

2 large zucchini, chopped
1 cup fresh or frozen peas, thawed
1 cup diced celery
1 avocado, peeled, seeded, and cut in quarters
¼–½ cup coconut water, depending on desired thickness
¼ cup fresh lemon juice
2 cloves garlic, chopped (to taste)
1 tsp. sea salt
1 tsp. fresh thyme
1 tsp. turmeric
Dash cayenne pepper
¼ cup chopped raw pistachios or almonds

Process zucchini, peas, celery, avocado, coconut water, lemon juice, garlic, salt, thyme, turmeric, and cayenne pepper until smooth. Pour into four bowls, and top each with 1 tablespoon of chopped pistachios or almonds. Serve cold if you want to retain all the vitamins and enzymes. If you desire a gently warmed soup, you can heat on a very low setting until just slightly warm. Serves 4.

Creamy Spinach Soup

I love spinach! It's a good source of iron, so it's a great food for people like me who are typically a bit low in iron. This is an easy, simply yummy soup that satisfies!

½ cup filtered water (add more as desired to get the consistency you wish)
2 cups spinach, chopped
½ avocado, peeled, seeded, and cut into quarters
1 rib celery, chopped
1 tsp. cumin
1 tsp. cayenne pepper
2 cloves garlic, chopped
Pinch sea salt
Pumpkin seeds for topping (optional)

Place all ingredients in a high-powered blender and blend until creamy. If desired, top with pumpkin seeds. Serve cold. Serves 2.

MENU PLAN FOR BREAKING THE FAST

Breakfast on the first day after your fast ends
Choose from the following:

+ Green smoothie

+ Fresh fruit

+ Fresh vegetables

Lunch
Choose from the following:

+ Vegetable salad with olive-oil-and-lemon-juice dressing

+ Vegetable soup (no dairy)

+ Steamed vegetables

Dinner
Choose from the following:

+ Vegetable salad with olive-oil-and-lemon-juice dressing

+ Vegetable soup (no dairy)

+ Steamed vegetables with quinoa

You may have seeds and ground nuts. Avoid grains except quinoa or sprouted buckwheat.

Eat no animal products at all the first day after your fast. Otherwise you could experience stomachaches and other digestive issues.

On the second or third day (depending on how long you have fasted), you can add in fish and/or an egg.

Chapter 8

THE DANIEL FAST MENU PLAN

Fasting makes you happy! Just as hunger makes you enjoy food more, so fasting is the spice of life and of food, especially when you are allowed to eat and dance again!
—St. Basil the Great

Also known as the Lenten fast or vegan fast, the Daniel fast eliminates animal products from your diet, along with sugar, alcohol, coffee, and junk food. Though there are a few other variations of this fast, they are mostly the same food plan.

This fast is a plant-based diet, which many proponents of health recommend. This type of diet has been life-changing for many people. It is typically a twenty-one-day fast based on Daniel's twenty-one-day fast in the Book of Daniel—hence the name. Though you don't have to fast for twenty-one days, it is highly recommended. Many people do this fast for forty days or more.

The Daniel Fast Menu Plan

There are seven soup and stew recipes and seven main-course recipes that follows, along with seven salad recipes. You can mix them up for your twenty-one-day program. You can try all the recipes or choose some of your favorites and repeat them. If you decide to fast for more than twenty-one days, you can get creative. On the Internet you'll find new vegan recipes to include in your menu planning. I encourage you to also include fresh juices and smoothies with your vegan foods because they offer many health benefits. See the recipes offered in chapter 7.

Start your day

Drink 8 ounces of purified water to start your day. It will flush your liver.

Next up

Drink a cup of hot water and lemon with a dash of cayenne. This will get your liver moving in the morning. Also, lemon is thought to cleanse the digestive tract.

Breakfast

Choose your recipe.

Midmorning pick-me-up

You may have fresh juice or a small snack, such as nuts or seeds.

Lunch

Choose your recipe.

Midafternoon rejuvenator

You may have a small snack, such as veggie sticks and hummus, or fresh juice.

Dinner

Choose your recipe.

Evening calming tea

Drink chamomile or chamomile lavender tea (or any other favorite herbal tea).

BREAKFAST RECIPES

Chia Breakfast Pudding

Chia-seed pudding is an easy overnight recipe. Soak chia seeds overnight to allow them to swell up like tapioca. Leave the seeds soaking in a bowl on the counter, covered with a tea towel or cheesecloth. This will create a creamy pudding with a unique texture. Add matcha green tea for an energizing breakfast pudding.

Fabulous Gluten-Free Pancakes

Our local Coeur d'Alene Michael D's Eatery offers my favorite Paleo pancakes. Since they don't share their famous pancake recipe, I've tried to replicate it. This is fairly close.

½ cup coconut flour
1 tsp. baking powder
½ tsp. sea salt
3 Tbsp. organic virgin coconut oil, melted
1 Tbsp. raw honey or coconut nectar
Egg replacer (equal to 3 eggs)
⅔ cup almond milk
1 tsp. vanilla extract
½ tsp. orange or lemon zest
Organic virgin coconut oil for frying pancakes
Maple syrup or coconut nectar, to serve for the topping

In a large bowl whisk together coconut flour, baking powder, and salt.

In a medium-sized bowl whisk together coconut oil, honey, egg replacer, almond milk, vanilla, and orange zest. Pour wet mixture into flour mixture and fold to combine, breaking up any large lumps. Melt oil on griddle or in pan until hot but not smoking. Pour batter in about ¼-cup measurements onto the griddle or pan. When you see bubbles in the batter and you lift one end and see it is golden brown, flip the pancakes. Check the center of a pancake in about 3–4 minutes for doneness. Pancakes should have no moist centers and be cooked all the way through.

Serve with butter or ghee (clarified butter) and maple syrup or coconut nectar, or put fresh fruit on top. Serves 2.

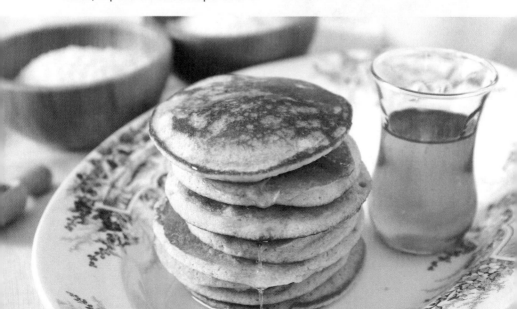

Nut-and-Seed Morning Smoothie

The combination of omega-3 fatty acids, high lignan content, and mucilage gums in flaxseeds makes this an excellent anti-inflammatory food.

10 raw almonds
1 Tbsp. raw sunflower seeds
1 Tbsp. chia seeds
1 Tbsp. sesame seeds
1 Tbsp. flaxseeds
1 pineapple or 1 cup unsweetened juice
1 cup chopped parsley
½ cup almond milk
½ tsp. pure vanilla extract
1 Tbsp. protein powder (optional)
6 ice cubes

Place the nuts, seeds, and pineapple juice in a bowl. Cover with a tea towel or cheesecloth and let it sit on the counter overnight.

Place the nut-and-seed mixture with the juice in a blender and add the parsley, milk, vanilla, protein powder (if using), and ice cubes. Blend on high speed until smooth. This drink will be a bit chewy because of the nuts and seeds. Serves 2.

Note: To kill molds, add 1 teaspoon ascorbic acid to juice, then add nuts and soak overnight.

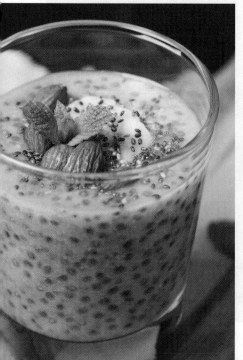

Sprouted Buckwheat Cereal

Buckwheat is known to improve heart health by lowering cholesterol and blood pressure.

Soak 2 cups of buckwheat groats in purified water overnight in a bowl set on the counter and covered with a tea towel or cheesecloth. The next day rinse them in a colander very well. Buckwheat groats have a lot of starch, so you'll want to rinse that away. Leave them in the colander overnight, covered with a tea towel. The next day you will have sprouts. Store them covered in the refrigerator. Take out what you wish for breakfast. I like to serve them with almond milk, ground almonds, and cinnamon. This is a delicious, enzyme-rich breakfast. Enjoy!

Overnight Soaked Muesli[1]

This is a great recipe to make with kids, especially since all the prep happens the night before and it's easy to finish quickly in the morning.

8 cups organic rolled oats
½ cup flaxseed, whole or ground
2 cups unsweetened currants
2 cups chopped nuts of choice, toasted
1 tsp. ground cinnamon
3–4 cups almond or coconut milk, to cover oats
2 apples
Fresh berries (optional garnish)

Put all dry ingredients into a large glass bowl or gallon bag to combine.

The night before you want to eat your muesli, put your desired portions of the oat mixture into a bowl and cover with almond or coconut milk. Grate ½ apple per person. Stir in immediately to keep apple from discoloring. Cover and place in the fridge overnight.

In the morning when you're ready to eat it, add more plant milk to taste. Great served with fresh berries. Serves 4–6.

Cherie's Awesome Green Smoothie

Research has identified more than forty-five different flavonoids in kale. With kaempferol and quercetin at the top of the list, kale's flavonoids, antioxidants, and anti-inflammatory benefits help us avoid chronic inflammation and oxidative stress.

1 avocado, peeled, seeded, and cut in quarters
1 cup baby spinach
2 kale leaves
½ cucumber, peeled and cut in pieces
Juice of 1 lime
1 Tbsp. green powder of choice (optional)
2–3 Tbsp. ground almonds (optional)

Combine all ingredients in a blender and blend well until smooth. Sprinkle ground almonds on top as desired. Serves 2.

Amaranth Pumpkin Porridge[2]

Amaranth is one of the "super grains" like quinoa, boasting a full nutrient panel and lots of protein. Here it's paired with pumpkin to make a rich and creamy breakfast porridge.

   1 cup dry amaranth
   ½ tsp. nutmeg
   1 tsp. cinnamon
   ⅓ cup shredded coconut flakes
   1–2 Tbsp. coconut sugar
   1 Tbsp. pure maple syrup
   2 Tbsp. organic virgin coconut oil
   ½ tsp. sea salt
   1 cup pumpkin puree
   2 ½ cups almond milk
   1 cup water (Omit if making "cakes"; recipe follows.)

Preheat oven to 400 degrees.

Bring all ingredients to a simmer over medium heat, stirring to combine (this takes about 10 minutes). Once the mixture comes to a low boil, turn off heat and cover with a tight-fitting lid or foil. Place in the oven.

Bake for 45–60 minutes. Use a hot pad to remove pot from the oven and stir well after removing, as liquid will sit on the top. Serve immediately, or cool and reheat in the morning.

You can reheat in a glass or ceramic dish in the oven at 425 degrees for 25 minutes for a hands-off way to enjoy a seasonal hot breakfast. Serves 4.

To make amaranth breakfast "cakes":

Follow the previous recipe, but omit the water and reduce the almond milk to just 2 cups. Cool the mixture completely in the fridge. In the morning pan-fry ¼ cup of this mixture in coconut oil over medium-high heat, pressing down to form little "cakes." Brown 2–3 minutes on each side, and drizzle with a little pure maple syrup. If the cakes fall apart, try adding 1 tablespoon of ground flaxseed and ½ cup gluten-free flour. Enjoy! Serves 4.

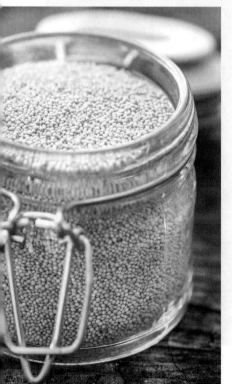

SALAD RECIPES

Benefits of Arugula

With its spicy flavor arugula adds a lot of zip to a salad. But that's not all it's up to! It's known to be cleansing for the blood, skin, and liver.[3]

One of its unique cleansing properties is to counteract the destructive effects of heavy metals, particularly in the liver. A member of the cruciferous vegetable family, arugula is rich in detoxifying antioxidants. It also sports an abundance of flavonoids, phytonutrients that are known to help prevent cholesterol from sticking to the arteries, thus lowering blood pressure and quelling inflammation. One study found that it could also help in fighting gastrointestinal ulcers.[4]

"A research team studying the natural health benefits of arugula discovered that it could be associated with fighting gastrointestinal ulcers, possibly through the many antioxidants it contains. Other studies have linked it to relief from gastric ulcer and psoriasis, as well as protection from skin, lung, and mouth cancers."[5]

Arugula Spinach Blueberry Detox Salad

1 cup arugula leaves
1 cup baby spinach
½ cup blueberries
1 small shallot, thinly sliced
2 Tbsp. cilantro leaves, chopped
2 Tbsp. mint leaves, chopped
2 Tbsp. basil leaves, torn
Juice of 1 lime
½ tsp. minced ginger
½ tsp. pink Himalayan salt
½ tsp. thinly sliced red chile or pinch of red pepper flakes
2 Tbsp. extra-virgin olive oil
2 Tbsp. toasted cashews, roughly chopped
2 Tbsp. pomegranate seeds
Pinch sesame seeds
½ avocado, sliced (optional)

Toss together arugula, spinach, blueberries, shallot, and fresh herbs in medium bowl. In a small bowl, whisk together lime juice, ginger, salt, red pepper, and olive oil. Pour dressing over greens. Sprinkle the cashews, pomegranate seeds, and sesame seeds over the top. Arrange the avocado slices on top, if using. Serves 2.

Donna's Zucchini Salad

"Several preliminary animal studies show potential anti-inflammatory protection from summer squash for the cardiovascular system and also for the GI tract."[6]

6 small zucchini, spiralized into noodles
1 small red onion, sliced
1 pint organic cherry tomatoes
1 green bell pepper, chopped
1 orange bell pepper, chopped
½ cup black olives
12 oz. marinated artichoke hearts, drained
Fresh chopped parsley as garnish

Homemade Italian Dressing

½ cup apple cider vinegar
¼ cup extra-virgin olive oil
½ Tbsp. garlic powder
½ Tbsp. onion powder
½ Tbsp. Italian herbs
½ tsp. Dijon mustard
½ tsp. dried basil
¼ tsp. ground black pepper
¼ tsp. sea salt
4–5 drops stevia

Dressing instructions:

In a small mixing bowl, whisk together all ingredients well to combine. Let it sit, sealed and refrigerated, for at least twenty-four hours before using so the herbs can infuse. Shake well before using.

Salad instructions:

Gently combine zucchini noodles with the dressing. Toss in remaining ingredients. Adjust seasoning as needed. Serves 4.

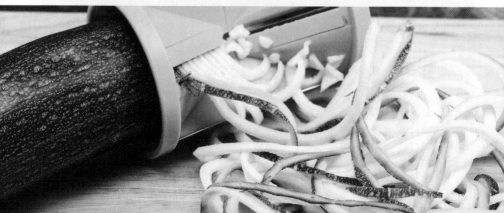

Carrot Radish Pumpkin-Seed Herb Salad

¼ cup extra-virgin olive oil, divided
1 cup raw pumpkin seeds, shelled
½ tsp. ground cumin
3 Tbsp. fresh lemon juice
1 tsp. coconut nectar or local raw honey
¼ tsp. freshly ground black pepper
1 tsp. sea salt, or to taste
2 pounds carrots, peeled, shaved into lengthwise ribbons with a
    vegetable peeler
1 bunch radishes (about 10), thinly sliced on a mandolin or with a sharp
    knife
4 cups (packed) herb mix, such as parsley, cilantro, dill, mint, tarragon,
    and/or basil
½ cup chopped chives

Heat 1 tablespoon of oil in a medium skillet over medium heat. Add pumpkin seeds and cumin and cook, stirring, until lightly toasted and fragrant, 4–5 minutes. Transfer to a plate and season with salt; cool.

Whisk lemon juice, sweetener, pepper, and ¾ teaspoon salt in a medium bowl until sweetener dissolves. Whisk in the remaining 3 tablespoons of oil until emulsified.

Toss carrots and radishes with dressing in a large bowl, and fold in herbs, chives, and half the pumpkin seeds. Top salad with remaining pumpkin seeds. Taste and season with salt and pepper, if necessary.

Sesame Kale Salad With Apple[7]

2 cups apple, sliced or shredded
1 clove garlic, minced
6 cups kale, chopped into bite-size pieces
1-inch-piece ginger, minced (optional)
1 tsp. sea salt
2 Tbsp. lemon juice
1 Tbsp. extra-virgin olive oil
½ Tbsp. sesame oil

Combine all ingredients in a large bowl. With clean hands massage the vegetables as if you are squeezing water out of them. Work the vegetables at least 15 times.

After 10 minutes, use a plate to hold the vegetables in the bowl, and tilt to drain the excess liquid into the sink. Work the vegetables another 15 times. If you prefer a saltier or more pickled salad, repeat the process 1–2 more times.

Enjoy many variations on the theme! Serves 4.

Asian Salad

Bean sprouts contain a significant amount of protein and fiber.

2 zucchini, sliced into strips with a vegetable peeler or mandolin
2 large handfuls bean sprouts, about 2 cups
¾ cup chopped nuts (suggest almonds or cashews)
1 red or yellow bell pepper, sliced into strips
4 green onions, diced
½ cup fresh chopped cilantro
Juice from one lime
1 Tbsp. extra-virgin olive oil
½ tsp. Celtic sea salt

Toss all ingredients together in a bowl until well coated. Serves 2.

DIY Salad With Avocado and Chickpeas With Lemon-Tarragon Dressing[8]

DIY means "do it yourself." This is where the magic of salads happens: improvising in your kitchen with the produce you have to make an on-the-fly fresh salad as a stand-alone meal or side dish. Think outside the lettuce box—chop up anything colorful and fresh for your salad, and experiment with fresh herbs to really brighten things up. Chop vegetables in bite-size pieces, especially if they are sturdy vegetables, such as beets or carrots. Anchor your salad with avocado and chickpeas to make it a meal-in-one.

Here is a starter list of ingredients for salad making. I encourage you to find even more ingredients to make your salads magical!

Apples	Ginger
Arugula	Jicama
Asparagus	Kale
Avocado	Mustard greens
Beets	Nectarines
Bok choy	Nuts/seeds
Carrots	Peaches
Celery	Pears
Cooked beans	Radicchio
Cooked chickpeas	Radish
Daikon	Scallions
Dandelion greens	Strawberries
Fava beans	Swiss chard
Fresh herbs (basil, mint, cilantro, rosemary)	Turnips
Garlic	Watercress

Lemon-Tarragon Vinaigrette

"Tarragon has long been used as a digestive tonic because it aids in the production of bile by the liver."[9]

¼ cup fresh lemon juice
½ tsp. lemon zest
½ tsp. Celtic sea salt, or to taste
¼ tsp. freshly ground black pepper, or to taste
1 large clove garlic, pressed
¾ cup extra-virgin olive oil
2 Tbsp. fresh tarragon, or 1 Tbsp. dried

Combine all ingredients except the oil and tarragon, and mix well. While whisking, drizzle in oil very slowly in a steady stream until an emulsion is formed. Add tarragon and mix well.

Broccoli Pomegranate Salad

"Johns Hopkins scientists have discovered that broccoli, which contains a unique chemical called sulforaphane (fights malignant cells in the body), also has the ability to detoxify the body of cancer-causing chemicals before they get a chance to promote cancer."[10]

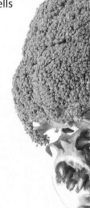

1 lb. broccoli (2 small heads)
1 ½ lb. carrots, peeled
1 cup pomegranate seeds
½ cup pumpkin seeds, toasted

Avocado Dressing

2 ripe avocados
¼ cup fresh lemon juice
2 tsp. sea salt

Chop the broccoli heads, and peel the stems of the broccoli and break into small pieces. Place in a food processor fitted with a chopping blade, and pulse until small pieces remain. Set aside in a big bowl.

Next, using the grater attachment, grate the carrots. Set aside with the broccoli. Add the pomegranate seeds and toasted pumpkin seeds and toss together.

Rinse the food-processor bowl, and place back on the base with the chopping blade to make the dressing. Peel the avocados and remove the pit. Place all dressing ingredients in the food processor and blend until smooth. Toss dressing with the salad and serve.

You may refrigerate for a few hours before serving. Serves 4.

SOUPS AND STEWS

Very Veggie Green-Bean Soup

Green beans are an excellent vegetable for the pancreas.

3 Tbsp. olive oil or organic virgin coconut oil
2 medium yellow onions, diced
2 ribs celery, diced
3 cloves garlic, minced
3 large handfuls green beans, trimmed
1 quart vegetable stock
1 cup almond flour
4 large chard leaves or other dark leafy greens, roughly chopped
¼ cup chopped parsley
Juice of 2 lemons
1 tsp. sea salt
Pinch of ground pepper

Heat oil in a large saucepan over medium-low heat. Add onions and celery and cook until vegetables have softened and turned golden in color, stirring occasionally. Add garlic and sauté for 30 seconds. Add green beans, stir well, and then add stock and all remaining ingredients. Simmer 30 minutes. Serves 4.

Spicy Lentil Soup With Delicata Squash

Sweet-dumpling and delicata squash are great sources of beta-carotene and vitamin C.

1 medium delicata squash or sweet-dumpling squash
2 Tbsp. extra-virgin olive oil
1 onion, finely chopped
1 tsp. sea salt, divided in half
3 carrots, chopped in small pieces
3 celery ribs, chopped in small pieces
½ cup fresh orange juice (optional)
1 tsp. curry powder
½ tsp. ground cumin
½ tsp. ground turmeric
½ tsp. ground coriander
½ tsp. ground cinnamon
Pinch red-pepper flakes
8 cups organic vegetable broth
1 cup dried green lentils, rinsed
1 cup packed kale, stemmed and chopped

Preheat oven to 350 degrees.

Place squash on a cookie sheet and bake for about 15 minutes or until the squash is tender enough to cut easily. Remove from oven and cool. When it is ready to handle, peel, seed, and cut into 1-inch cubes. (I've found this is the easiest and safest way to cut up hard squash.)

Heat olive oil in soup pan over medium heat. Add onion and ½ teaspoon salt; sauté until onion is translucent, about 5 minutes. Add carrots, celery, and squash. Adjust salt as needed. Sauté until the vegetables are tender, about 5 minutes. Add seasonings and other ½ teaspoon sea salt. Add 1 cup of broth. Add lentils and stir. Cook until liquid is reduced by half. Add the remainder of the broth and the orange juice. Increase the heat and bring to a boil. Then decrease the heat to low, cover, and simmer until lentils are tender, about 30 minutes. Adjust seasoning. Add kale and cook another 5 minutes. Serves 6.

Brown Lentil Rhubarb Soup

"While many believe milk is the best calcium source, one cup of cooked rhubarb contains just as much, and it's actually much better for you."[11]

1 bunch chard, chopped
2 Tbsp. olive oil or organic virgin coconut oil
1 onion, chopped
2 carrots, chopped
2 ribs celery, chopped
1 Tbsp. minced fresh ginger
3 cloves garlic, minced
1 tsp. cumin
½ tsp. turmeric
Sea salt and pepper to taste
1 cup brown lentils, rinsed and drained
4 cups vegetable broth
1 lb. rhubarb, trimmed and chopped
½ cup currants
Chopped cilantro, for serving

Remove leaves from chard stems; chop stems. Slice leaves and put aside.

Heat oil in a large soup pot over medium-high heat. Add onions, carrots, and celery. Sauté until veggies begin to soften, about 7–8 minutes. Stir in chopped chard stems, ginger, garlic, cumin, and turmeric; cook until fragrant, about 2 minutes. Season with salt and pepper.

Add lentils and broth, and bring to a boil. Reduce heat and simmer for 30 minutes. Stir in rhubarb, chard leaves, and currants. Simmer until rhubarb and lentils are tender, about 10 minutes more. Top with cilantro. Serves 4.

Spiced Eggplant and Sweet Potato Stew

This stew is one delicious way you can get more eggplant into your diet. Here's an important reason why you would want to eat this vegetable: "When laboratory animals with high cholesterol were given eggplant juice, their blood cholesterol, the cholesterol in their artery walls and the cholesterol in their aortas (the aorta is the artery that returns blood from the heart back into circulation into the body) was significantly reduced, while the walls of their blood vessels relaxed, improving blood flow."[12]

2 Tbsp. extra-virgin olive oil or organic virgin coconut oil
1 eggplant, cut in large chunks
1 medium onion, chopped
1–2-inch-chunk ginger root, peeled and grated
1 Tbsp. garam masala
1 can (15 oz.) garbanzo beans
1 large sweet potato, peeled and cut into chunks
1 large can (28 oz.) stewed tomatoes
1 can (14 oz.) coconut milk
Sea salt and pepper to taste

In a large soup pot, heat the oil over medium heat and sauté the eggplant until golden and slightly soft. Remove eggplant with slotted spoon and set aside.

Sauté the onion, ginger, and garam masala for about 5 minutes, or until the onion is soft. Drain garbanzo beans and add to the pot with the remaining ingredients except the eggplant. Bring to a boil and simmer for about 30 minutes, or until the sweet potato is soft. Then add eggplant and simmer for another 30 minutes.

Adjust seasoning to taste and serve with rice. I especially like red or green rice. Serves 4.

Pumpkin Curry Soup

"In scientific tests, pumpkin has been shown to reduce blood glucose levels, improve glucose tolerance and increase the amount of insulin the body produces."[13]

1–2 Tbsp. extra-virgin olive oil or organic virgin coconut oil
1 onion, chopped
2 garlic cloves, chopped
1 Tbsp. grated ginger
3 tsp. curry powder
½ tsp. ground cumin
¼ tsp. ground cardamom
1 can (15 oz.) unsweetened pumpkin puree
1 can (14 oz.) coconut milk

½ cup vegetable broth
½ cup fresh apple juice
1 tsp. sea salt
Dash black pepper
¼ cup roasted pumpkin seeds for garnish

Heat oil in a large soup pot over medium heat. Add the onion, garlic, and ginger, stirring frequently until the onion is soft. Add the spices and stir. Cook for 1 minute. Add the pumpkin and coconut milk. Whisk in the broth and apple juice. Increase the heat and bring to a boil. Reduce heat to low and simmer for 5 minutes. Stir in salt and pepper. Transfer to a blender and puree. Spoon into bowls and add pumpkin seeds. Serves 4.

Lemon-Herb White-Bean Soup

Beans are an inexpensive source of protein that can help lower your cholesterol.

1 package (20 oz.) Great Northern beans
8 cups water
2 Tbsp. olive oil or organic virgin coconut oil
1 cup onions, diced
2 cloves garlic, minced
2 Tbsp. fresh lemon juice
1 large carrot, chopped
½ tsp. thyme
½ tsp. basil
½ tsp. rosemary
½ tsp. celery powder
2 tsp. sea salt

Place rinsed beans in a soup pot and cover with the water. Allow beans to soak overnight, or 8 hours. Then drain.

Pour 8 cups of fresh water over the beans, and turn the heat on high. Bring to a boil.

While beans are coming to a boil, place oil in small skillet and sauté with the onions and garlic for about 5 minutes, or until the onion is soft. Add the onion-garlic mixture to the soup pot along with the lemon juice and carrot. Simmer, covered, for 1½ hours, making sure the beans are always covered with water. Check beans for tenderness. Add the herbs and salt. Adjust seasoning to taste. Serves 4.

Bone Broth

There's a South American proverb that says, "A good broth can raise the dead."

4–5 grass-fed beef bones, chicken bones, or any mixture of bones from
　wild or pasture-raised, healthy animals; if using beef bones, choose
　meaty beef shank. You can find such bones at natural markets and at
　some grocery stores that carry grass-fed products.
Purified water
1 Tbsp. raw apple-cider vinegar
1 carrot, chopped
¼ onion
1 clove garlic
Sea salt and pepper

Place bones into a large soup pot or electric cooking pot. You need only a few bones to make a great broth. Fill your pot with filtered water to cover all the bones completely. Add the vinegar, carrot, onion, and garlic. Season with salt and pepper to taste. Add fresh herbs if you have some. Turn your heat on low for the soup pot, or set your electric cooking pot on low. Simmer for 24 hours. I put my soup pot in the oven on 200 degrees overnight. Poultry bones can simmer as long as 24 hours, and beef bones can simmer for up to 48 hours.

When the pot is cool enough to handle, pour the broth through a sieve into containers. You can use tongs to pick the bones out first. Store in the refrigerator. It should keep for 5–7 days, or freeze for later. Skim fat layer off the top, if it forms.

MAIN DISH RECIPES

Burdock Root With Vegetables

1–2 Tbsp. olive oil or coconut oil
½ medium onion, chopped
1 burdock root, chopped
1 carrot, chopped
1 small beet, chopped
2 Jerusalem artichokes, chopped
1 cup broccoli, chopped (or another green vegetable, such as nettles)
2–3 cloves garlic, chopped
2–3 sprigs parsley
1 Tbsp. lemon juice

Sauté onion in olive oil or coconut oil. Sauté the onion until translucent and then add the rest of the vegetables with the chopped garlic. When the vegetables are lightly cooked, add chopped parsley. Salt and pepper to taste. Sprinkle with lemon juice. Serves 2.

Sweet Potato–Black Bean–Quinoa Burgers With Lemon-Tahini Sauce

Sweet potatoes are rich in beta-carotene. Current studies show that if you include some fat with them—a minimum of 3–5 grams— you will significantly increase your uptake of beta-carotene with that meal.

2–3 medium sweet potatoes
1 can black beans (15 oz.), rinsed
¾ cup cooked quinoa
½ cup red onion, chopped
½ cup chopped walnuts
1 Tbsp. Dijon mustard
1 tsp. ground cumin
½ tsp. sea salt
½ tsp. ground pepper
2 Tbsp. organic virgin coconut oil or extra-virgin olive oil

Bake the sweet potatoes at 350 degrees for about 45 minutes or until tender. Remove from the oven and slice in half. When they are cool enough to handle, scoop the flesh into a bowl. Add the beans and quinoa, and mash together with a fork. Mix in the rest of the ingredients, except the oil.

Heat a large skillet over medium heat and add the oil. Shape the mixture into approximately 12 patties. Cook patties for about 5 minutes on each side or until they form a crispy golden crust.

While patties are cooking, make Lemon-Tahini Sauce.

Lemon-Tahini Sauce (or Dressing)

This makes a delicious salad dressing as well as sauce. For salad dressing, add a little more water.

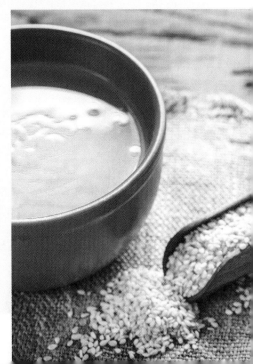

¼ cup tahini
¼ cup water
¼ cup fresh lemon juice

Mix tahini, water, and lemon juice in a blender until creamy. Gently warm in a saucepan. Top each burger with tahini sauce.

Herb and Chickpea Croquettes With Rosemary-Walnut Pesto, and Cider-Braised Greens and Green Beans[14]

Herb and Chickpea Croquettes

"Participants in a recent study reported more satisfaction with their diet when garbanzo beans were included, and they consumed fewer processed food snacks during test weeks in the study when garbanzo beans were consumed."[15]

This is one of my favorite dishes of all time. Not only is this recipe delicious; it's satisfying.

1 cup chickpeas (garbanzo beans), cooked
⅓ cup extra-virgin olive oil, for batter
1 cup cooked quinoa
½ cup shallots, diced
2 garlic cloves, minced
½ cup celery, diced
½ tsp. dried oregano
½ tsp. sea salt
1 Tbsp. Dijon mustard
½ cup almond meal or gluten-free breadcrumbs
⅓ cup all-purpose gluten-free flour or oat flour
¼ cup coconut or grapeseed oil, for pan frying

Pulse the chickpeas and olive oil together in a food processor, or mash in a bowl with a tool. Combine all ingredients in a bowl, and add the mashed chickpeas and oil. Taste for flavor and let sit 10 minutes. If dough seems dry, add more olive oil until you can easily form a ball in your hand. Form into balls no bigger than 2 inches in diameter.

Heat a pan with ¼ cup oil over medium heat until hot. Fry croquettes 2 minutes per side, and if needed place on a baking sheet and finish cooking in the oven at 350 degrees until browned and crispy on the exterior but not dry, about 5–10 minutes. Replenish oil as needed, changing out oil if brown bits form. (Scrape oil into a bowl lined with a strainer so you can use the oil once more for frying.) Serves 4.

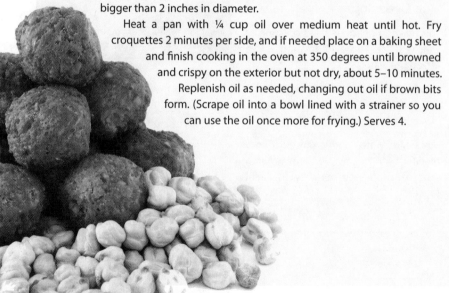

Rosemary-Walnut Pesto

This is a winter pesto recipe—try it with kale in place of parsley! Come summer, substitute basil or cilantro for the rosemary (about ½ cup) to keep this recipe current with the season.

1 bunch parsley
2 sprigs rosemary
1 clove garlic
1 cup walnut
⅓ cup chickpeas or white miso
½ tsp. sea salt, or to taste
1 cup extra-virgin olive oil
Juice of half a lemon (optional)

Combine the first six ingredients in a food processor, slowly pouring in the olive oil. Adjust flavor and consistency as desired. Add the juice of half a lemon for a bonus alkalizing kick! Yields 2 cups.

Cider-Braised Greens and Green Beans

1 cup apple cider
¼ cup organic virgin coconut oil
1 tsp. sea salt
1 head collard greens, destemmed and chopped
2 cups green beans, destemmed and chopped
1 Tbsp. apple-cider vinegar

Heat apple cider in a medium-size skillet over high heat. Allow the cider to reduce at a rapid boil for 5 minutes or until reduced by half. Add oil and salt, and stir to combine. Add collard greens, green beans, and apple-cider vinegar, and continue to boil. Lower heat to low and braise for 5–7 minutes. Taste and serve. Serves 4.

Quinoa With White Beans and Roasted Peppers

Quinoa is a great grain to include in a vegan diet because it is high in protein.

2 cups water
1 cup quinoa
½–1 tsp. sea salt
¼ tsp. ground black pepper
1 cup roasted red peppers, cut in 1-inch pieces
¼ cup extra-virgin olive oil
½ cup fresh lemon juice (about 2 large lemons)
½ cup pine nuts
1 cup fresh mint leaves, torn

1 carrot, halved lengthwise and thinly sliced crosswise
1 can (15 oz.) white beans, such as Great Northern beans, drained and
     rinsed

In a medium saucepan bring the water to a boil and add the quinoa, salt, and pepper. Cook about 15 minutes or until most of the water is absorbed. Remove from the heat. Cover and let stand for about 5 minutes, or until all the water is absorbed.

While the quinoa is cooking, roast the peppers. While the peppers are roasting, add the oil and lemon juice to a small skillet, and over medium heat toast the pine nuts, gently shaking the skillet occasionally, for about 5 minutes, until fragrant and just starting to turn brown. Stir in the carrots and white beans; warm for 5 minutes. Transfer to the quinoa.

Fold in the roasted peppers and mint. Adjust the seasoning to taste. Serve warm. Serves 6.

South-of-the-Border Lettuce Wraps

2 ripe avocados
3 tomatoes, diced
½ jalapeño pepper, diced
2 Tbsp. yellow onion, diced
3 cloves fresh garlic, minced
¼ cup fresh cilantro, chopped
Kernels cut from one ear raw corn
2 tsp. fresh lime juice
6–8 large lettuce leaves

In a medium-sized bowl, mash the avocados. Add the remaining ingredients and stir until well mixed. Spread 2–3 tablespoons of this mixture onto lettuce leaves, and wrap. Serves 6–8.

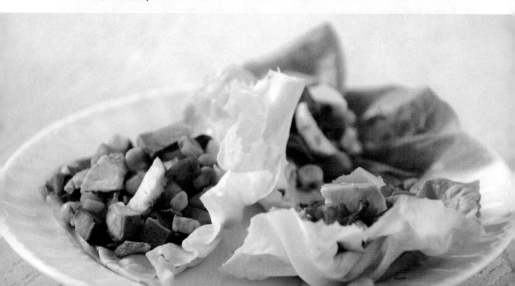

Squash and Arugula Enchiladas[16]

Delicata squash is my favorite in this recipe. It features yellow skin with green stripes on an oblong shape. A ¾-cup portion of it contains just 30 calories, so it's a great choice if you are wanting to lose weight. It's a good source of vitamin C and carotenes. Adding arugula or watercress gives you an example of combining cooked and living food.

2 delicata squash or 1 acorn squash or about ¼ butternut squash (other
    winter squash, sweet potatoes, or yams can be substituted)
1 cup brown rice, cooked
½–1 cup chopped arugula or watercress
4–6 tortillas (sprouted whole grain, spelt, or gluten free)
1 Tbsp. organic virgin coconut oil
Salt and pepper to taste

Bake the delicata squash in a preheated oven set at 400 degrees for 30 minutes or until tender but not soft. If you add water about an inch deep to the baking pan, it will cook faster.

While the squash is baking, cook the rice. When the squash is tender, remove from the oven and cut in half. Scoop out the seeds and peel. (If you're using delicata and the skin is tender, you don't need to peel.) Cut the squash into chunks and mix with rice; add seasoning to taste and set aside, keeping it warm.

In a large skillet, heat the oil. Heat the tortillas one at a time until warm and slightly browned. (Be careful not to overcook, or they will get crisp and won't roll into an enchilada.) Spoon 2–3 tablespoons of the squash-rice mixture into the center of each tortilla, and spread from one end to the other. Add arugula to the top of that mixture and roll each side toward the center. Serve hot. Serves 4–6.

Carrot Sauce With Asparagus and Fresh Peas Over Brown Rice

This is one of my favorite recipes. It's very fresh and is made with a carrot-juice sauce and summer vegetables.

1 cup brown rice or quinoa
1 ½ cups carrot juice (about 8–11 carrots)
½ cup raw cashews
2 Tbsp. white or yellow miso
1 lb. fresh asparagus
½ cup fresh or frozen peas
2 scallions, chopped
¼ cup marinated sun-dried tomato halves, thinly sliced
2 cloves garlic, pressed
3 Tbsp. finely chopped fresh basil

Heat water and add the rice or quinoa when boiling; cook according to directions.

Meanwhile, juice the carrots and reserve 1 ½ cups carrot juice.

In a blender or food processor combine the carrot juice, cashews, and miso; blend on high until the cashews are no longer gritty and the mixture is smooth and creamy.

Snap off the tops of the asparagus. Cut the tender upper portion into 1-inch pieces.

In a medium-sized skillet, combine the carrot juice mixture and asparagus. Bring to a boil and then reduce the heat to a simmer, stirring occasionally for 2–3 minutes. Add the peas and simmer until the asparagus is just tender, about 2 minutes. Add the scallions, sun-dried tomatoes, and garlic, mixing well; simmer for 1–2 minutes. Remove the sauce from the heat.

Divide the rice or quinoa into four portions. Top each portion with about ¼ of the sauce, and sprinkle chopped basil on top of each portion. Serves 4.

Easy Lentil Skillet Dinner

This recipe is easy and delicious. I never have leftovers.

2 cups steamed French green lentils (you can buy these pre-made)
2 cups cooked quinoa
2 Tbsp. organic virgin coconut oil or extra-virgin olive oil
1 cup chopped onions
2–3 carrots, chopped
2 cloves garlic, minced
2 Tbsp. chopped ginger
2 lb. fresh spinach, washed and dried
1 small zucchini, chopped
1–2 tsp. Celtic sea salt

Prepare lentils according to instructions. Prepare quinoa according to instructions.

In a large skillet, melt coconut oil; add onions and carrot and sauté for about 5 minutes or until onion is translucent and carrots are tender. Turn to low heat, add garlic and ginger, and sauté for about 3 minutes. Add zucchini and salt; sauté for 3–4 minutes. Place cooked lentils in skillet and mix well. Add spinach to the top and cover with a lid. It will steam. Allow about 4–5 minutes, or until spinach is just slightly wilted. Serve over cooked quinoa. Serves 3–4.

SNACK RECIPES

Kale Chips[17]

1 bunch kale
¼ cup fresh lemon juice
¼ cup apple-cider or coconut vinegar
¼ cup extra-virgin olive oil
½ tsp. Celtic sea salt
2 tsp. garlic, minced or pressed (optional)
Pinch cayenne pepper

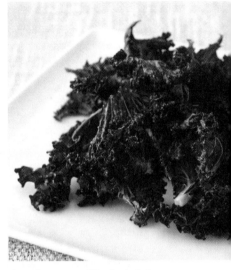

Wash the kale, and then cut it into 3-inch-long strips and set aside to dry. Add lemon juice and vinegar to a bowl. Very slowly pour in the olive oil by dripping it in from a distance of about a foot above the bowl while whisking continually. This will create an emulsion in which the oil is well combined with the other ingredients and won't separate as easily.

Then stir in the sea salt, minced garlic (if using), and cayenne. Dip the kale in the marinade. Shake off excess marinade, and place kale pieces on dehydrator sheets. Dehydrate for 7–8 hours at 105–115 degrees or until crisp. (Chips will get smaller as they dehydrate.) Makes 40–50 chips.

These chips are so delicious, I'll bet you won't have any left to store!

Onion Rings[18]

3–5 onions (yellow, white, or Walla Walla sweet)
¼ cup fresh lemon juice
¼ cup apple-cider or coconut vinegar
¼ cup extra-virgin olive oil
½ tsp. Celtic sea salt
2 tsp. garlic, minced or pressed (optional)
Pinch cayenne pepper

Cut onions into thin slices and set aside. Add lemon juice and vinegar to a bowl. Very slowly pour in the olive oil by dripping it in from a distance of about a foot above the bowl while whisking continually. This will create an emulsion in which the oil is well combined with the other ingredients and won't separate as easily.

Then stir in the sea salt, minced garlic (if using), and cayenne. Add the onion slices to the emulsion, and marinate for several hours.

Shake off excess marinade so that onion rings are not dripping with marinade. Place onion rings on dehydrator sheets, and dehydrate for about 7–8 hours at 105–115 degrees or until crisp. Makes about 40 rings.

Dehydrated Zucchini Chips

Slice zucchini into thin rounds, and sprinkle with a little Celtic sea salt, as desired. You can also sprinkle your favorite seasoning on them. Place zucchini slices on dehydrator sheets, and dehydrate for about 12 hours at 105–115 degrees or until crispy. These are surprisingly sweet and delicious. Makes about 12 chips per zucchini.

Vegan Cheese

This is great on brown rice or dehydrated crackers. It also makes a great dip for veggies.

> 2 cups raw macadamia nuts
> ¾ cup nutritional yeast
> 1 ½ tsp. onion powder
> ¾ tsp. garlic powder
> ½ tsp. sea salt
> 3 Tbsp. water
> 2 tsp. fresh sage, finely chopped (or substitute ½ tsp. dried sage)
> 1 handful parsley, minced

Soak the macadamia nuts overnight.

Drain off the excess water and place the nuts, nutritional yeast, onion powder, garlic powder, salt, and water in a food processor fitted with the blade attachment. Process until creamy. Add more water as needed. Be careful, though—too much water, and the mixture will become mushy. Fold sage into the nut mixture.

Roll mixture into a 10-inch log, and then roll the log in minced parsley. Serve with veggie sticks or crackers. Serves 6.

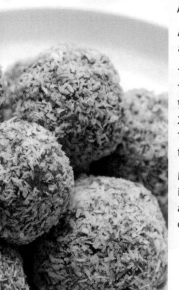

Almond Butter Balls[19]

Almond butter is a healthier choice than peanut butter and equally delicious.

16 oz. almond butter (crunchy or creamy)
1 tsp. cinnamon
¼ tsp. stevia or ¼ cup coconut nectar (or to taste)
2 cups rolled oats or oat flour
1 cup unsweetened shredded coconut flakes or finely chopped nuts

Mix almond butter, cinnamon, and sweetener together in a bowl. Use oats as they are, or blend them until they assume a powder-like texture (or use oat flour). Add oats to the nut butter-sweetener mixture and mix until

combined, working with hands. Adjust consistency if necessary.
Roll batter into small balls. Wet hands often to prevent mixture from sticking to hands. Roll balls in coconut flakes or chopped nuts. Chill and eat! Makes 40 balls.

Notes: This recipe yields a lot, so you can freeze the balls and grab a few when you need a snack or are craving something sweet. It's worthwhile to make them all at once and freeze them or keep them in the fridge for up to ten days.

THE GARDEN OF EDEN FAST

A version of the Daniel fast, the Garden of Eden fast is made up of only perennial plants—the types of plants that would have grown in the Garden of Eden. Though there are still a lot of foods you can eat, your selection is more limited. Choose from the following list. Many recipes in the Daniel fast will also fit for the Garden of Eden fast. This is a list of perennial plants available today. It is believed that in the Garden of Eden there were more fruits and nuts with a few veggies such as watercress.

Perennial vegetables

Artichoke (Jerusalem, also known as sunchoke)	Sweet potato
Asparagus	Tree cabbages/tree collards
Radicchio	Watercress
Rhubarb	Yams
Spinach (Ceylon, Sissoo, or New Zealand)	

Perennial Fruits

Apples	Lemons
Apricots	Limes
Avocado	Nectarines
Blackberries	Olives
Cherries	Oranges
Currants	Peaches
Dates	Pears

Fig	Persimmon
Goji berries	Plums
Grapes	Raspberries
Huckleberries	Strawberries
Kiwi	

Perennial legumes

Beans (winged or Scarlet Runner)

Perennial cereal grains

Wild rice

Perennial nuts

Almond	Pecan
Chestnut	Pistachio
Hazelnut	Walnut
Macadamia	

Perennial herbs

Alfalfa	Lemon balm
Basil	Mint
Chives	Onions (potato onions, shallots, Egyptian onions, Japanese bunching onions, Welsh onions, or Chinese leeks)
Fennel	Oregano
Garlic	Parsley
Ginger	Rosemary
Horseradish	Sage
Lavender	Thyme

Chapter 9

THE SPIRITUALITY OF FASTING

with Fr. John Calbom

Fasting is the food of the soul.
—ST. JOHN CHRYSOSTOM

MARCH 6, 2016, will go down in my personal history book as one of the more challenging days of my life. My hard drive crashed. And it didn't just stop working—everything was lost. Then I discovered that my Time Machine backup had failed in recent attempts to back up my work. Actually two years of work was lost, including the initial work on this book.

It was Sunday, the day after my husband's stepfather's memorial service. We were in Gig Harbor, Washington, at his sister's, getting ready to drive home to Couer d'Alene, Idaho. I flipped open my laptop so I could pull up e-mails to go through as we drove. The screen was frozen. I shut it down and turned it back on. I'd done that drill before. But this time it gave me a weird message and nothing worked.

I scheduled a Genius Bar appointment at the Apple Store as we headed down the freeway; they'd always fixed everything in the past. We went straight there before going home.

And I learned the bad news.

I felt numb the rest of the day—as if I'd lost a dear friend.

As I sat in the quiet of my office that evening, I asked the questions I always do in challenging moments: *What is the meaning in this? What can I learn?* Then it dawned on me. The hard drive crashed on Sunday. Hadn't I struggled for quite a while to just rest on the Sabbath, or the day of rest, as it's also known? For Christians the day of rest is Sunday; for Jews it runs from sundown Friday to sundown Saturday.

> Remember the sabbath day by keeping it holy.
> —EXODUS 20:8, NIV

Marci Alborghetti quotes a Jewish woman in *Daily Guideposts 2016*: "[The Sabbath is] a twenty-four-hour period during which we admit we are not as important as we think, and God's world goes on without us."[1] How important did I think I was, and how important was my work? I went to church faithfully, but that was where the rest ended. The remainder of the day I worked. I always thought I had so much to do—e-mails to answer, a newsletter to write for my Monday e-blast, and usually a book to write...on and on it went. Typically I'd start my workdays by answering e-mails, many times before prayer, and end my day doing the same just before I fell into bed, exhausted. My life felt out of order most of the time, and especially on my day of rest.

According to Abraham Joshua Heschel the Sabbath is "a palace in time which we build."[2] As one writer says, "It's not a day of rest before work; you work in order to experience this day of elevation....Even successful lives need these sanctuaries."[3] My Sabbath day of rest took on new meaning. What a message; what a lesson! I now do my very best to start each day with prayer and devotional reading before anything else.

This led me to think about fasting in light of the busyness and drivenness we all get trapped in from time to time—or all the time. In *Wisdom From the Monastery* Peter Seewald says, "When we fast we let everything go—all the things that we dragged around with us, all the things that clung and stuck to us. The weight under which we were collapsing was our own."[4]

From time to time we all need to fast from work, busyness, overload, crazy-making behavior, and overachieving. We all need a day of rest and a life that is in order with intervals of rest. This is part of the spirituality of fasting, part of an ordered life.

But resting is even more crucial when we embark on a period of fasting. This is the time to slow down and let some things go. The e-mails will wait, as well as the callbacks. All the "must-dos" can stack up for a little while. You can still get your work done, but more time should be devoted to prayer, meditating, reading, and relaxing. (Yes, relaxing is permitted in the twenty-first century!) This is the time to quiet your heart and mind and listen to your soul.

LETTING GO OF DRIVENNESS

What does it mean to be driven? The online version of *Merriam-Webster's Dictionary* says that *driven* means "having a compulsive or urgent quality."[5]

I had been driven for quite some time. I think it all started when a friend told me I should make sure before I made an appearance on a certain program that my website was working well and could handle lots of traffic. I needed a good e-mail capture system to grow my newsletter list and to answer people as soon as possible so I wouldn't lose them. My friend said a friend of hers had done the same program I would be on and had a big response, but her website couldn't handle it and went down. She lost all the potential people who would have come to her from that show. This lodged in my brain like the rudder of a ship and steered my turbo-charged life from that moment on.

In fact, I don't think I ever turned off. I did that show and more shows, hit the trail running, and never looked back—until my life seemed to crash with my hard drive. A couple weeks later my website was hacked and crashed too. Then it crashed three times after that. Everything came to a screeching halt—right during Lent, the church's season of fasting. I had to ask myself, "What have I been doing? What has all of this been about?" Drivenness is now at the top of my list of things I need to fast from.

Do you also need to fast from drivenness? From busyness? From filling your life's plate too full? Do you need to fast from what you put into your mind regularly? From what types of reading you do? What kinds of TV programs you watch? How much of your time is devoted to it? Letting all this go from time to time is part of the spirituality of fasting—the healing of our lives.

Ask yourself these three questions:

+ What is my intention for fasting?

+ What do I want to accomplish with a fast?

+ What do I hope will change in my life and transform in my soul, as well as my body, as I fast?

For Your Consideration

Now is the time to examine your life. Are there areas in which you can fast spiritually, let go, and find renewal? Though this list is not exhaustive, consider these areas and add your own:

+ Living from the false self, or not being who you really are

+ Being consumed with getting ahead, or focused on accumulating things

+ Demonstrating injustice toward others, or treating others unkindly (in religious traditions, fasting is a time of joy and showing special kindness to others)

+ Being dishonest, or not being honest with yourself and others at all times

+ Being self-indulgent, and not just with food (fasting will unveil food indulgences and addictions though)

+ Being consumed with self-interest, or lacking concern about the needs of others

+ Seeking pleasure or living for good times and the good life

+ Not giving when you see people in need (again, in religious traditions, fasting is a time of almsgiving)

+ Lacking peace, being irritable, and feeling agitation

Spiritual Terra Firma

Firma means "solid." And since I want this chapter on the spirituality of fasting to be built on solid ground, I've asked my husband, Fr. John Calbom, to write the remainder of this chapter. A Russian Orthodox priest (yes, they can marry!), a psychotherapist, and a cardio biofeedback specialist, Fr. John is the best source I know to address the spirituality of fasting. Between his degree in theology and his practical experience as a priest in a church that fasts periodically throughout the year, he's my terra firma for this part of the fasting journey. You're in good hands as you enjoy the rest of this spiritual journey.

A RETURN TO THE SOURCE OF LIFE

After Adam and Eve disobeyed God, their first instinct was to try to separate themselves from their Maker to be their own gods and hide from Him (Gen. 3:8–10). In other words, they embraced the illusion that they could live separately from their Creator. Not only that, but they also hid *behind* the things of creation, namely the trees of the garden: "And they heard the sound of the LORD God walking in the garden in the cool of the day, and Adam and his wife hid themselves from the presence of the LORD God among the trees of the garden" (v. 8). God then called Adam and Eve out of hiding. He made garments to cover over their nakedness (v. 21) and promised to send a redeemer (v. 15).

Ever since Adam and Eve, our first parents, chose to be the gods of their own lives, mankind has attempted to live separate from God, using the things of creation to hide from Him. But being separated from the source of life—or believing the illusion of separateness—is not a good place to be since it means that our survival lies in our own hands. Consider just a few of the pathologies that arise out of a sense of separateness from the source of life:

+ To be separated from the source of life is to assume the burden of our own survival. Living in a state of survival activates the reptilian part of the brain, with the result that people are seen as objects to be used or threats to be avoided.

+ To be separated from the source of life means that it's up to us to use the things of this culture (food, sex, money, recreation, other people) for our emotional, psychological, and mental survival.

+ To be separated from the source of life is to desperately need others to validate us in order to give us the security we cannot generate for ourselves. Relationships thus become a minefield of stress since we are expecting from others what only God can provide.

+ To be separated from the source of life is to continually fear death and to try to mitigate death's sting through maladaptive behaviors, such as emotional eating and surviving at the expense of other people.

+ To be separated from the source of life means that the burden of giving meaning to our lives, or demonstrating to others that our lives have worth, depends on us.

+ The sense of separateness from the source of life leads us to use the things of this culture as surrogate forms of life. We try to improve the quantity or quality of our life and thus mitigate the sting of our approaching death through hoarding good things to ourselves.

These are just a few examples of how we lose our spiritual path through separateness from God. Every day we experience the results of not being immortal, of the death principles working in us. As David Fontes observed, our first parents "went from *life eternal* to *life survival* because of their sin of disobedience."[6] But the good news is that we don't need to stay in this disordered state. Through the Incarnation and saving death of Christ mankind has been given back what was lost in the garden, namely eternal life (John 10:10). Many people think eternal life simply means going to heaven when you die. While going to heaven is part of the picture, eternal life also means plugging back into the source of life *right now* in the present.[7] We can begin today to experience the security and peace of being united with God, of plugging back into the source of life.

But what does this mean in practice? For one, it means that instead of hiding from God as Adam and Eve did, we can let God do what He specializes in doing: taking care of us. Remember that after God called Adam and Eve out of hiding, He made skins to cover their nakedness and later provided a means of restoration of relationship with Him. We too can return to God in all our vulnerability and let Him take care of our needs. Instead of hiding behind the things God has made, looking to the things of creation for our mental, emotional, and spiritual survival, we can trust God to meet our needs. We can relax and let go, released of the burden of trying to be our own God. As we do this, God can help us work on the toxicity of the soul we've built up through spending so much time in survival mode.

When everything seems to be going wrong for us, it's easy to slip back into that survival mode. When we feel pain, uncertainty, vulnerability, fear, and confusion, or when we remain hampered by the consequences of past failures, it's easy to believe that God is an incompetent CEO. When other people mistreat us, abuse us, and speak negatively about us, it takes a lot of faith to believe that God will help us to use everything for our best.

During difficult times the temptation is to feel as if we are separate from God and, hence, that our mental, emotional, and psychological survival depends on us. If we give in to this impulse—and assume control of our own survival instead of trusting God—then all manner of maladaptive behaviors emerge.

When we are lonely or lack healthy relationships, the temptation is to survive by forming disordered connections with people through control, competition, flattery, possessiveness, lust, or enabling behaviors. When other people hurt us, misuse us, or abuse us, the temptation is to survive by hardening ourselves, becoming invulnerable, or adopting various defense mechanisms. When we hurt ourselves through our own actions and thoughts, the temptation is to survive through denial or through imposing our own narratives on reality that make us feel better. When we believe lies about ourselves that make us feel worthless, the temptation is to assert ourselves through behaviors such as competition, control, manipulation, or aggression. When we are bored or when our lives seem to lack a sense of purpose, the temptation is to survive by filling up our emptiness with shallow pleasures such as food, e-mails and texts, TV, computer games, or social media. However innocent these pleasures may be in themselves, they can never satisfy the heart's longings. As survival mechanisms, these maladaptive behaviors and emotions feed the illusion that we can exist separately from God and that the source of life can be found in the things of creation rather than in the Creator.

The two most primal survival mechanisms are those connected with the body—food and sex. Once mankind was separated from the source of life, the body began gravitating toward food and sex in a heightened way since it is through these things that we survive, both individually and as a species. Even when we're not hungry, our stomach and brain still send us the message "I need that food right now to survive." When we respond to our body's urges, we eat more than we need, resulting in overeating and obesity.

Similarly, if a man is walking down the street and sees a beautiful woman, his body will often cry out, "I need her to survive!" Whether or not he has the opportunity or intention to gratify this lust, and even if it is only a passing feeling, the body is sending a very clear message: *I am separate from my Creator and thus require the things of creation for my survival.* This leads to the overindulgence of the sexual appetite through disorders such as pornography, immorality, and lust. As with Adam and Eve in the garden, what seems "pleasing to the eye, and also desirable" (Gen. 3:6, NIV) leads to the sense of separateness, whereby we move away from God and hide behind created things (v. 8).

When we fast, we have the opportunity to come out from hiding and get to the root of our toxic thinking, emotions, and actions. By choosing to go without certain foods during a period of fasting, we are making a powerful proclamation that our survival does not depend on the things of this culture. When our body is crying out for food, sex, or entertainment and we choose to turn to God instead of our appetites, we are proclaiming that our survival depends on God alone. Accordingly periods of fasting are opportune times for us to seek life from the Creator rather than the creation. They are times to stop trying to meet our needs without God. Fasting is a time to plug back into the source of life, get out of survival mode, and trust God.

Fasting is a journey toward wholeness and spiritual healing. This is an opportunity to reestablish the right relationship among your spirit, soul, and body. However, spiritual healing does not come automatically simply by giving up certain foods. Rather, we can turn to God and seek a *spiritual* fast as well as a *physical* fast.

WHY A SPIRITUAL FAST?

Americans spend inordinate sums on their bodies. From personal-care products to hairstyles to fitness services, we spare no cost. But what if we were as attentive to our inner lives as we are to our outer lives? What if we were as devoted to the health of our souls as we are to our physical health and well-being?

These are questions that fasting encourages us to ask. Fasting is certainly good for our bodies, yet the physical advantages are secondary to the spiritual rewards. When we fast, we are invited to take a step back from our fast pace of life and attend to our inner life. Fasting invites us to activate our own inner physician, to temporarily stop focusing on satisfying bodily wants and to focus on the needs of our souls.

Below are some of the spiritual benefits derived from periods of fasting. Some of these benefits can be experienced immediately, whereas others only emerge after years of regular fasting routines:

+ Fasting helps to slow down the mind so we can focus on the things of the spiritual world. At the same time mental functions are enhanced.

+ Seasons of voluntary deprivation remind us of all we have to be grateful for. During periods of fasting we are often enabled to better appreciate some of the blessings we might otherwise have taken for granted.

+ The hunger and tiredness that accompany fasting (especially at the beginning) offer us a chance to identify with the poor and needy and to experience Christ's blessing on those who are "poor in spirit" and who "mourn" (Matt. 5:3–4).

+ The struggle involved in fasting is a chance to follow the apostle in disciplining our bodies to bring them "into subjection" (1 Cor. 9:27). This develops valuable skills that can be used to overcome various physical temptations, such as lust and overeating.

+ When the body's functions are slowed down through lack of food, we are better enabled to rise above our fast-paced lives and the tyranny of the urgent. This gives us the opportunity to attend to our mental and emotional well-being through fasting from toxic thoughts and feelings. (For more about this, see chapter 10.)

+ Our culture is constantly telling us that we need various things or experiences in order to be happy. Fasting invites us to challenge this narrative. It's a time to ask, "Is God enough?"

+ Fasting underscores the truth that there is an interconnection between body and soul. It reminds us that what we do in our bodies has spiritual implications.

+ Fasting is associated with being humble. If done with a right attitude, fasting can lead to an increase in humility.

+ Fasting enables us to see ourselves more clearly. Bernhard Müller said, "People who fast can see things more clearly and can, when necessary, change their ways more easily and chart a new course. . . . The small, difficult steps of fasting allow us gradually to consider new possibilities for life in the future. How far these new experiences can carry the person who is fasting varies according to the individual."[8]

+ Fasting is a powerful testimony to the fact that food does not have to control us; we can control it.

Fasting offers us the opportunity to realign ourselves with God by letting go of false gods. It often isn't until we begin fasting that we are able to recognize the false gods of our lives that control us. As Richard Foster observed, "More than any other Discipline, fasting reveals the things that control us. This is a wonderful benefit to the true disciple who longs to be transformed into the image of Jesus Christ. We cover up what is inside of us with food and other things."[9]

One false god that often controls us is food. Because food is necessary for our physical survival, it's easy to begin thinking that food itself is what gives us life, that food enables us to flourish, that food satisfies our soul. In short, it's easy to treat food as a god. Accordingly we think we have to satisfy our desire for food at all costs, even if it means sacrificing our health and well-being. Though few of us would think of food as a god, we often act as if it is.

Our idolatrous valuation of food fits comfortably with our culture's obsession with the body. Through things such as billboards, television commercials, and various types of advertisements we are told in countless ways that happiness and satisfaction are the result of having our bodily needs met. As Susan Gregory observed, "In a culture of great affluence it's easy to yield to the ways of the world...the self-centered ways of our society. 'If I want it I buy it. If I am hungry for it [I] eat it.' And that mind-set has led millions of people into a life [of] debt, disease, and obesity."[10] The lie that true joy comes from satisfying our bodily needs lies at the root of comfort eating and most of our society's other addictions and disorders.

Fasting helps to turn this around, underscoring God's words: "Man shall not live by bread alone" (Deut. 8:3; see also Matt. 4:4). When indulgent behaviors and ways of thinking have become habitual, the discipline of fasting calls us to a higher path. It challenges us to connect with the ultimate source of life, which is not food but God Himself. Fasting is a time to begin a new journey without food to satisfy our emotional needs.

None of this is to imply that food is intrinsically bad. Throughout history food is treated as a gift—a good thing that God created. But even good things can become problems when they become overindulgences. The fast is a time to be reminded that our desire for food and other joys of this world are mere trifles. This is a point that John Piper brought out in the introduction to his excellent book *A Hunger for God: Desiring God Through Fasting and Prayer*:

> The greatest enemy of hunger for God is not poison but apple pie. It is not the banquet of the wicked that dulls our appetite for heaven, but endless nibbling at the table of the world. It is not the X-rated video, but the prime-time dribble of triviality we drink in every night. For all the ill that Satan can do, when God describes what keeps us from the banquet table of his love, it is a piece of land, a yoke of oxen, and a wife (Luke 14:18–20). The greatest adversary of love to God is not his enemies but his gifts. And the most deadly appetites are not for the poison of evil, but for the simple pleasures of earth. For when these replace an appetite for God himself, the idolatry is scarcely recognizable, and almost incurable.[11]

It's in the Book

The Bible is full of examples of people connecting with God through fasts. Consider just a few:

- Moses fasted for forty days and nights before receiving the tablets of the Law from God (Exod. 34:28).
- When King Jehoshaphat learned that a great multitude of enemies was coming against the people of Judah, he "set himself to seek the LORD, and proclaimed a fast throughout all Judah" (2 Chron. 20:3).
- The inhabitants of Nineveh avoided impending disaster with a period of fasting (Jonah 3:5–10).
- The prophet Elijah fasted for forty days and nights in the desert to prepare for an important mission (1 Kings 19).
- After Queen Esther learned of a plot that Haman had devised to murder all the Jewish people living in Persia, she instructed her people to observe a strict fast. They abstained from all food and water for three days and nights (Esther 4:16). God honored their time of fasting and prayer and delivered them.

- Before Jesus began His public ministry, He fasted for forty days. The fast strengthened Him to resist temptation and prepared Him for His ministry (Matt. 4:1–11).

- When Christ's disciples asked Him why they couldn't cast a demon out of a child, He told them, "This kind does not go out except by prayer and fasting" (Matt. 17:21).

- The centurion Cornelius had the truth of God revealed to him through the apostle Peter after a time of prayer and fasting (Acts 10:30).

FASTING IN THE EARLY CHURCH

Fasting played an important part in ancient Judaism. In particular, fasting was a way for faithful first-century Jews to remember that while they were living in their ancient homeland, they were still in a state of spiritual exile, awaiting the promised deliverer.

At the time Jesus was born, the Jewish temple had men and women dwelling in it who devoted their lives entirely to prayer and fasting. This was a precursor to what would later become the Christian tradition of monasticism. We read about one such person in Luke's infancy narrative. When the baby Jesus was eight days old, Mary and Joseph took Him to be circumcised in the temple, according to the custom prescribed by Moses. While in the temple Mary and Joseph met an aged woman named Anna who "served God with fastings and prayers night and day" (Luke 2:37).

The very earliest documents from the Christian era show that Christians continued the Jewish practice of fasting. The Book of Acts makes many references to the Christian practice of fasting. For example, it was only after a period of fasting that the Holy Spirit gave instruction to set apart Paul and Barnabas for missionary work (Acts 13:2). During their missionary journey to appoint elders in the various churches, Paul and Barnabas "prayed with fasting" wherever they went (Acts 14:23).

One of the earliest surviving Christian texts outside the New Testament is a treatise called *The Didache*, or *The Teaching of the Twelve Apostles*. This anonymous work, which scholars believe dates from the first century, was used for the instruction of catechumens (those who were preparing for baptism). It instructs Christians to fast twice a week, on Wednesdays and Fridays, a practice that has continued to this day in many of the oldest branches of Christendom.[12]

Among the other earliest Christian texts there are frequent references to fasting. In her survey of fasting in the early church Joan Brueggemann Rufe mentions just some of the many occasions in which early Christians would fast:

> These early Christian texts show Christians fasting to prepare for baptism, to mourn and commemorate Jesus' death...to better resist temptation, to obtain revelation, as part of their observance of stations, in response to persecution, and to care for the poor and address community needs and support community goals.[13]

Fasting didn't come easy for the early Christians. In fact, fasting is often mentioned in Scripture by the phrase "afflict your souls" (Lev. 16:29–31; 23:27–32; Num. 29:7; 30:13). But though fasting was a hardship, the early Christians gladly embraced it as a way to apply the Pauline injunction, "We must through many tribulations enter the kingdom of God" (Acts 14:22).

In the early days of the church Christians didn't need much reminder that the spiritual life is hard work. After all, they were being killed left, right, and center. "Many martyrs are daily burned, confined, or beheaded, before our eyes," wrote the church father Clement of Alexandria (c. AD 150–c. 215).[14] The persecution of Christians culminated in a decree by the emperor Septimius Severus (145–211) in 202 that made it a criminal offense for a person to convert to Christianity.[15]

Despite this increasing opposition the church continued to grow, producing both converts and martyrs in great number. It wasn't that the church was growing in spite of persecution; it was growing *because* of persecution. By a type of strange spiritual logic the more the church suffered, the stronger it became. This led the church father Tertullian (160–220) to remark in his *Apologeticus*, "The oftener we are mown down by you, the more in number we grow; the blood of Christians is seed."[16] As Christianity expanded, the Roman authorities devised more creative and hideous ways to torture Christians, hoping to force them to renounce their faith in Christ. To gain courage in the face of so much hardship, the early Christians fasted and prayed.

Then the unthinkable happened. The emperor became a Christian. In 313 the emperor Constantine issued the Edict of Milan, which officially stopped the persecution of Christians. Around the same time, Constantine publicly proclaimed himself to be a Christian. Suddenly it became popular to be a believer. Constantine died in 337, but his legacy continued. The emperor Theodosius, who ruled from 379 to 395, went even further and made Christianity the official state religion. And Christianity became easy.

Those who could remember the days of persecution knew that while it was a blessing to no longer be hunted and killed, it was also a challenge. It was now possible to be lax and indulgent. One could worship Christ and still live a comfortable life, following after the idols of power, prestige, and bodily comforts. In short, the church was in danger of becoming a lot like the culture around it. Hadn't Jesus said that the way to the kingdom of heaven was through poverty of spirit (Matt. 5:3), mourning (v. 4), and persecution (vv. 11–12)?

It was at this point in church history that fasting took on an even greater significance. Fasting became a way for Christians to voluntarily deny themselves and thus to experience the type of spiritual growth that comes from hardship. Fasting and other self-imposed ascetic training became a way for Christians to reject the life of ease and reintroduce struggle into the spiritual journey. As St. John Chrysostom (c. 349–407) said in a sermon on Hebrews, "Mortify your body; crucify it, and you will receive the martyr's crown. What the sword did for the martyrs, let your own will do for you."[17]

Fasting for Your Mind

"All the purely mental powers of man improve while fasting. The ability to reason is increased. Memory is improved. Attention and association are quickened. The so-called spiritual forces of man—intuition, sympathy, love, etc.—are all increased. All of man's intellectual and emotional qualities are given new life. At no other time can the purely intellectual and aesthetic activities be so successfully pursued as during a fast."[18]

Throughout the third century many Christian men and women moved to the Egyptian desert to engage in fasting and other spiritual practices. One such man was Anthony the Great (251–356), a wealthy landowner who sold all his possessions and moved to the desert to embrace a life of fasting and prayer. St. Anthony's diet consisted only of bread, salt, and water, and he would eat no more than once a day, sometimes going three or four days without his daily meal.

St. Anthony never intended to become famous. However, the church father Athanasius of Alexandria (c. 296–373) wrote a book, *Life of Anthony*, which became a best seller. This widely read book caused countless men and women to go into voluntary exile in the desert to imitate St. Anthony and spend their lives seeking God. Through the practice of frequent fasts these desert dwellers were able to experience the same spiritual benefits that had previously been available to the persecuted church.

Paradoxically, by embracing poverty and fasting and rejecting self-indulgence, these desert men and women were able to excel in gratitude to God for His spiritual gifts. Cornelius Plantinga Jr. observed how these desert dwellers revealed the strange spiritual logic that going without food leads to greater gratitude and a heightened appetite for God:

> Self-indulgence is the enemy of gratitude, and self-discipline usually its friend and generator. That is why gluttony is a deadly sin. The early desert fathers believed that a person's appetites are linked: full stomachs and jaded palates take the edge from our hunger and thirst for righteousness. They spoil the appetite for God.[19]

Bernhard Müller described some of the spiritual activities that occupied these desert dwellers:

> The first hermits, or "desert fathers," were looking for three things in the desert: prayer, fasting, and solitude. Their dwellings were uncomfortable and cramped, their clothes were simple, they slept little, and ate simply and sparingly between periods of daylong

fasting. It is reported that these men battled "every day like athletes, and as a result succeeded in controlling their bodily need for food, achieving absolute poverty, true humility, and sanctification of the body."

...It was not unusual for people to consider their inner being as a real battlefield in which the greatest enemy was their own self will.[20]

As communities of prayer rose up in the desert, they gradually spread throughout the entire Christian world, making it possible for men and women to follow the example of Anna, who "served God with fastings and prayers night and day" (Luke 2:37). When the Western Roman Empire began to be overrun by barbarians in the late fourth century, these communities helped to preserve stability, maintain learning, and shine as beacons amidst the darkness.

Not only did monastic communities spread, but also church leaders who had been trained in the monasteries helped ordinary Christians begin ordering their lives through the disciplines of prayer and fasting.[21] At the same time, people were counseled not to go overboard in their zeal. For example, St. Antony warned that "there are some who weaken their bodies through fasting; they are far from God because they do not exercise moderation."[22]

Looking at the early church from the vantage point of our comfortable twenty-first-century lives, we may find it strange that so many men and women would choose to embrace this austere lifestyle. However, the early Christians teach us that hardships—whether through persecution, fasting, or some other means—are good for the soul. Through hardship God can strengthen our faith, working in our hearts patience, long-suffering, and a desire for the life to come.

In many parts of the world today to be a Christian is to invite persecution and even death. While we don't generally experience these hardships in the West, we do face other challenges. One challenge is that in living a life of ease and comfort, we can become complacent and apathetic. Fasting is a way to reverse this trend and remind ourselves that the spiritual life is one of discipline and spiritual work. Like the early

Christians who fled to the desert following the Christianization of the Roman Empire, fasting enables us to identify with those who suffer in other parts of the world.

ACTIVATING THE "INNER PHYSICIAN"

When Ron Lagerquist was eighteen, he abandoned his life as a drug addict and became a Christian. In the early years after his conversion Ron spent hours studying Scripture and singing songs to God on his knees.

By the time he was in his early twenties the cares of life had taken over, even though Ron was still a Christian. He tells how "slowly over time, a life of spirituality was replaced by busyness. Daily cares choked to death intimacy with my Father. It happened so slowly, I didn't even notice."[23] To fill the emptiness, Ron turned to junk food:

> A wiry teenage body transformed into an overripe pear. Prayer was replaced by eight different kinds of chocolate bars stockpiled in my drawer. Street Ministry was replaced with Saturday Night Hockey, supplemented by a large bag of salt and vinegar potato chips and candy coated peanuts, Bible reading substituted for a two-kilogram tub of butterscotch ice cream. My covert stash and I met regularly, intense moments of escape from intimacy gone dry. Not knowing it at the time, I had replaced the drug addiction of my early years with a different type addiction, junk food.[24]

After enduring thirteen years of "a slow spiritual ice age,"[25] Ron discovered fasting. By removing the props of junk food that had covered his emptiness, Ron was able once again to come face to face with himself. It was not easy. Regret and repentance marked the early days of his fast. But slowly, over time, Ron came back to life. He credits God's grace with reviving his spirit and prayer life. Eventually, he found himself moving toward others with increased compassion and love.

Ron said he experienced detox symptoms from too much caffeine, salt, hot dogs, and fries. There were days that he felt sick and headachy, had a foggy brain, and was emotionally out of sorts. But eventually the negative symptoms went away, and he was renewed.

What Ron experienced at the beginning of his fasting experience—confusion, turmoil, and depression—is typical. During a fast the body diverts the energy it would normally use for digestion (about 30 percent) and channels it into healing.[26] As the body's healing processes are initiated, toxins are released. That is why it is typical to have bad breath or to sweat when you fast, especially if you are fasting for the first time.

But just as physical toxins come to the surface so they can be eliminated, spiritual toxins also rise to the surface in a process that Dr. Buchinger has called "a kind of unraveling and loosening of a tensed-up spiritual structure."[27] Consequently, it is normal for fasting to make you feel worse before you begin feeling better. When fasting brings spiritual toxins to the surface, it is time to recognize the addictions, compulsions, and fears that may have previously been disguised to you.

What the Fast Reveals

"If pride controls us, it will be revealed almost immediately when fasting. David said, 'I humbled my soul with fasting' (Ps. 69:10). Anger, bitterness, jealousy, strife, fear—if they are within us, they will surface during fasting. At first we will rationalize that our anger is due to our hunger; then we will realize that we are angry because the spirit of anger is within us. We can rejoice in this knowledge because we know that healing is available through the power of Christ."[28]

"Passions," remarked the sixth-century monk Isaac of Syria, "are like dogs, accustomed to lick the blood in a butcher's shop; when they are not given their usual meal they stand and bark."[29] Be prepared for fasting to cause your passions to start barking. Sometimes a person who begins fasting will experience violent mood swings and bad dreams. Again, this is the soul's way of bringing unresolved issues to the surface so that you can deal with them. Bernhard Müller experienced this in a pilgrimage to a monastery in Germany, as recounted in the book *Wisdom From the Monastery*. He shares that the monk who was guiding him "explained to me that when fasting one undergoes not only a physical but also a spiritual detoxification."[30] He continues:

Bad dreams and mood swings were all signs that unresolved problems were being pushed up to the surface and required clarifica-
tion. I could now understand that fasting prevented disease in the
truest sense of the word: I could see not only how my body was
getting rid of toxins but also that how [sic] I was undergoing a
spiritual "spring cleaning."[31]

As the spiritual toxins come to the surface during the fast, we face an
important choice: either we can confront our inner demons and move
toward healing, or we can give in to the spiritual toxicity, becoming
cranky, irritable, and mean-spirited. In *The Diary of a Russian Priest*
Father Alexander Elchaninov tells a story that illustrates this point. A
critic of fasting commented to him that fasting caused their work to
suffer and the people to become irritable. The critic pointed out that
during Holy Week—the time when Russian Orthodox Christians
observe the strictest of fasts—people were more bad-tempered than at
any other time of the year. Father Alexander replied, "You are quite
right.... If it is not accompanied by prayer and an increased spiritual life,
it merely leads to a heightened state of irritability."[32]

Know the Symptoms

"It is well to know the process your body goes through in the course of a longer fast. The
first three days are usually the most difficult in terms of physical discomfort and hunger
pains. The body is beginning to rid itself of the toxins that have built up over years of poor
eating habits, and it is not a comfortable process. This is the reason for the coating on the
tongue and bad breath. Do not be disturbed by these symptoms; rather be grateful for the
increased health and well-being that will result. You may experience headaches during
this time, especially if you are an avid coffee or tea drinker. Those are mild withdrawal
symptoms that will pass though they may be very unpleasant for a time."[33]

THE RIGHT ATTITUDE

The year was 1570, and the tsar Ivan the Terrible was preparing to move
against his own people in Pskov, suspecting them of treason. Facing
the imminent slaughter of their entire community, the people of Pskov
gathered to pray during the first Saturday of Lent.

In the city of Pskov there dwelt a beggar named Nicholas who lived under the church bell tower. Though everyone called him "the Fool," Nicholas was known for his great wisdom. When he learned of Ivan the Terrible's plan to destroy the city, he tried to stop the tsar, but to no avail.

Ivan thought of himself as a spiritual man, so he accepted an invitation to visit Nicholas in his cell. (A cell is a small room used by a hermit or monk.) Upon Ivan's arrival, Nicholas offered the tsar a piece of meat.

"I am a Christian and do not eat meat during Lent," Ivan responded.

Nicholas replied, "But you drink human blood."

Convicted by Nicholas's words, the tsar ordered his men to turn back and leave the people of Pskov alone.[34]

This story illustrates the important point that fasting, in and of itself, is of no avail. To have value, fasting must be combined with faith and brotherly love. Jesus had some of His harshest words to say to the religious leaders of His own day who made a great show of their fasting while neglecting the weightier matters of the law (Matt. 6:16–18). Similarly Basil of Caesarea condemned the fourth-century hypocrites who would fast while slandering and criticizing their brothers and sisters. "You do not devour flesh," he said, "but you devour your brother."[35]

It's easy for us to fall into the same trap when we fast. The trap is to think we're earning spiritual favor while neglecting to show love. Fasting involves so much more than simply abstaining from food. Periods of fasting are times to be especially receptive toward God's grace and then to be a reciprocal of that grace to the people around us. Periods of fasting give us the opportunity to reevaluate what is important in our lives and to abstain from our passions, addictions, and indulgences. If we are abstaining from food but not abstaining from our typical busyness or addictions, such as shopping or the Internet, then our fasts have little spiritual value. As St. John Chrysostom observed, fasting "consists not in abstinence from food, but in withdrawing from sinful practices," adding, "Let not the mouth only fast, but also the eye, and the ear, and the feet, and the hands, and all the members of our bodies. Let the hands fast, by being pure from rapine and avarice. Let the feet fast, by ceasing from running to unlawful spectacles. Let the eyes fast, being taught never to fix themselves rudely upon handsome countenances."[36]

There is a Triodion (service book) that is read during the first week of Lent in the Eastern Orthodox churches that gets at the same point:

> As we fast from food, let us abstain also from every passion…
> Let us observe a fast acceptable and pleasing to the Lord.
> True fasting is to put away all evil,
> To control the tongue, to forbear from anger,
> To abstain from lust, slander, falsehood and perjury.
> If we renounce these things, then is our fasting true and
>   acceptable to God.
> Let us keep the Fast not only by refraining from food,
> But by becoming strangers to all the bodily passions.[37]

If not accompanied by the spiritual life—prayer, compassion, giving, forgiveness—fasting loses its spiritual value. Remember, as fasting brings spiritual toxins to the surface, we have a choice of addressing them or letting our passions master us.

The most common types of passions that emerge during a fast are those connected with disordered thoughts and emotions. That is why the following chapter will provide step-by-step techniques for detoxifying your mind and emotions and regaining control over what you think and how you feel. The good news is that you do not have to be a victim of toxic thinking and out-of-control emotions. You can fast from toxic thinking and toxic emotions and let them go for good.

Chapter 10

FASTING FROM TOXIC THINKING AND EMOTIONS

with Fr. John Calbom

> Fasting cleanses the soul, raises the mind, subjects one's flesh to the spirit, renders the heart contrite and humble.
> —Saint Augustine

ASTING IS A time to look at everything—not just what we eat and drink but also what we think and feel. I have been musing about this very thing as I look more in-depth at fasting and ask the question: What good does it do for us to avoid all the junk food, solid food, meat, dairy, sweets, alcohol, coffee, and sodas if we harbor toxic thoughts and emotions in our minds and hearts?

In the aftermath of the burglar attack that I shared with you in the introduction, I not only had severe physical injuries; I also experienced devastating inner wounds. In fact, the inner breaks in my being seemed far more shattering than the tears in my scalp, crushed discs in my neck, and shattered bones in my right hand. I called it my emotional tsunami. Suffocating pain stuck in the crevices of my soul. I sat on the floor in the corner of my bedroom one day, rocking back and forth, overcome by the inner torment and seriously thinking of escaping deep inside, where I could no longer feel the pain.

From a Psychology 101 class I had taken, I knew it was a catatonic state I was contemplating. I remembered my professor saying it was hard to get people out of that state once they got there. An inner voice whispered, "Hang on for one more day." And each day, I heard that voice again, as one day at a time turned into weeks and months.

Grace came into my life. I met three ladies—my kitchen angels, as

201

I called them—who prayed for me around a kitchen table once a week. Bit by bit, an emotion and thought at a time, I let go of toxic emotions and thoughts. It was my salvation from the complete destruction of my life.

At a Victims of Violent Crimes support group I learned that many victims of violent crimes such as the one I had experienced commit suicide. Instead of death I chose life. I chose it by letting go of the junk food of the soul, one small bit at a time. It was the most significant fast I'd ever undertaken, in many respects. I know I would not be here today, writing this section of my fasting book, were it not for this process of emotional and mental fasting I went through—a process of letting go.

Many people say they just can't let go of certain emotions and thoughts. They are so angry about the offenses committed against them—the loss, the abuse, the atrocity, the abandonment, the betrayal, the trauma, the hurt. Far worse things have happened to other people than what happened to me. Yet I know that the only path to life and freedom is letting go of the toxic thoughts and emotions that can hold us captive.

Holding on doesn't change the outcome. We may feel empowered for a moment…but we are not free when we're bound by destructive inner thoughts and feelings. We can be free even if we're imprisoned, maligned, abandoned, traumatized, or abused. I love the powerful words of Etty Hillesum, a Jewish woman born in Holland who lived in Nazi-occupied Amsterdam and was put to death at Auschwitz:

> This morning I cycled along the Station Quay enjoying the broad sweep of the sky at the edge of the city and breathing in the fresh, unrationed air. And everywhere signs barring Jews from the paths and open country. But above the one narrow path left to us stretches the sky, intact. They can't do anything to us, they really can't. They can harass us, they can rob us of our material goods, of our freedom of movement, but we ourselves forfeit our greatest assets by our misguided compliance. By our feelings of being persecuted, humiliated, and oppressed. By our hatred. We may of course be sad and depressed by what has been done to us; that is

only human and understandable. However, our greatest injury is one we inflict on ourselves.[1]

As I look back on my life, I think I've always had a wonderful life. (*It's a Wonderful Life* is one of my favorite movies of all time, in fact!) But other people might say it doesn't look so wonderful from their viewpoint. As I also mentioned in the introduction, my brother died at birth when I was two. I also contracted bulbar polio at two and nearly died. My mother was diagnosed with breast cancer when I was four and died when I was six. I lived with my maternal grandparents, and my dearly loved Grandpa John died when I was nine. I lost my father when I was thirteen, not to death but to a terrible tragedy that would take a chapter to tell. I went to live with an aunt and uncle the next year because my grandmother, at eighty-six, was too old to care for me any longer. A few years later she died. I was so sick in my late twenties with chronic fatigue and fibromyalgia that I could no longer work. I was attacked by the burglar a year after I recovered from those illnesses and was left for dead.

But has it been a life of pain and suffering? Quite the opposite, in my view. I share the words of St. Catherine of Siena: "All the way to heaven is heaven." It's all a choice. The vistas of our lives are up to us.

Fasting is your time to let all the harmful emotions and hurtful thoughts go—just as the song titled "Let It Go" from the movie *Frozen* says. You really can fast from this toxic stuff. Releasing it all usually comes not overnight but in small steps and stages. It's the old example of peeling the onion one layer at a time. Believe me when I say you can do it! It is freeing, restorative, and rewarding.

Rebecca Ondov shares a great analogy of letting go of hurtful emotions. She tells the story in *Guideposts* magazine of delivering a heavy roll of fencing wire to her friend Lou. It had taken a forklift to get the wire roll into her truck. How were they going to get it out of the truck, just she and her friend? But that wasn't her only burden that day. She felt as if a two-ton weight was rolling around inside her soul, just like that bail of wire in the back of her truck, because of a friendship that had gone off the rails.

Just then, she had a crazy thought: "Gun the accelerator and race toward the unloading spot; then slam on the brakes." That launched the wire roll right off the truck and onto the spot where Lou wanted it to be.

Rebecca felt as if her spirit said that was what she also needed to do with her broken friendship and the emotions pent up in her soul that were tearing her apart. She unloaded her burden to God, and gradually the hurt and broken friendship healed.[2]

Would that we could just "gun it" and let the hurtful emotions fly out of our souls in one quick projection, like that wire roll of Rebecca's! Sometimes we can, but mostly it takes patient persistence and work.

Fasting is an excellent time for you to do your work of the soul—*soul* meaning mind, will, and emotions.

Once again I place you in good hands with my husband, Fr. John, for the rest of this chapter and the fasting you can do to be fully free on the inside. My psychotherapist priest husband has dedicated his life to helping people break free of their burdens, their pent-up toxic emotions, and their inner wounds. He will guide you on your emotional and mental fasting journey too.

HOW TOXIC THOUGHTS AND EMOTIONS AFFECT YOUR BODY

We are not our thoughts and emotions. But if you have become accustomed to living in survival mode, then it is likely you have built up a residue of toxic thoughts, emotions, and habits. It is also likely that you are experiencing the effects of toxic thinking throughout your body.

Barbara Levine struggled with an inoperable brain tumor that led her to discover "seedthoughts" and "core beliefs" that link one's mind and body. In a book titled *Your Body Believes Every Word You Say* she traced common phrases such as "that breaks my heart" and "it's a pain in the butt" to underlying beliefs on which they are based and the symptoms they cause.[3]

Many of us don't recognize the underlying beliefs that our bodies believe or the messages that our brains are constantly sending throughout our systems. Physicist and psychologist Buryl Payne, PhD, explains the widespread power of our thought life throughout the entire body:

> We know that thoughts generated in the brain activate hormone secretions and stimulate other nerve centers within the body. Thoughts, coded as neural impulses, travel along nerve axons, activating muscles and glands similar to the manner in which telephone messages travel over wires in the forum of electrical signals. Experiments with the GSR, a biofeedback instrument, attached to fingers or toes clearly demonstrate that mental activity reaches into the extremities of the body.[4]

The notion that thoughts have physical ramifications may seem obvious to many. Have you noticed you have more energy and generally feel better when your thoughts are characterized by compassion, love, appreciation, and gratitude versus when your thoughts are obsessed with worry, bitterness, fear, or anxiety? Although we experience the physical effects of toxic thoughts and emotions every day, it has only been recently that the medical community has begun taking seriously the connection between thoughts, emotions, and physical health. In his foreword to *The Heartmath Solution*, Stephan Rechtschaffen, MD, said that "the body/mind split [is] so pervasive in medicine today," noting:

> We've separated the role of our thoughts and daily stresses from the effects that they produce in the physical body. Throughout their medical training, physicians are told of bacterial, metabolic, toxic, and other causes of physical illness, yet the relationship of our thoughts and emotions to effecting physical change is for the most part ignored. This has in large measure led to a medical model that can be dehumanizing, focusing solely on the specific physical manifestations of disease, thus losing sight of the whole person.[5]

Although the medical community is still dominated by a truncated approach to the human person, many practitioners are coming to recognize the need to focus on the whole person. In our book *The Complete*

Cancer Cleanse, I shared some of the groundbreaking medical research on how toxic thinking affects the body, including research showing that toxic thoughts and emotions are just as destructive to our health as poor food choices and polluted air.[6] Since we wrote that book, the scientific research has continued to advance. Many researchers are now suggesting that as much as 75–98 percent of illnesses may actually originate from our thought lives.[7] It is now clear that when we think negative thoughts, when we ruminate over bad memories, when we focus on negative emotions and fixate on what is wrong in our lives, we actually cause negative proteins to be released into the blood.[8]

By contrast, when we focus on positive things, when we let go of the things we can't control, when we have compassion for people who have hurt us or do things that are annoying, and when we focus on what is good in the world and in others, we can actually affect the makeup of our DNA and turn ourselves into healthier people.[9]

This isn't just theory. Cherie and I personally have witnessed the healing results of letting go of toxic thoughts and emotions. Many people who attend our juice-and-raw-foods wellness retreats have been helped by this process. Some who come are sick, while a few even suffer from life-threatening diseases. As we teach our retreatants how to let go of toxic thoughts and emotions, many people have found release from things that have plagued them for years, and we've seen many miracles. They let go of what's blocking them and what's keeping God's life-giving energies from reaching them. People have experienced release from toxic emotions and thoughts that have weighed them down for years.

Why do toxic thoughts and emotions have such an effect on the health of our bodies? One of the reasons is that thoughts and memories actually have a physical component to them and are stored in neurons inside the brain. That means that every thought you think, every memory you form, is located somewhere in the brain. In fact, the neurons that store our thoughts make up around 15 percent of all our brain cells.[10]

Now the really amazing thing about this is that when these thoughts and memories are toxic, the brain cells are unhealthy—they actually look different from healthy cells. In Dr. Caroline Leaf's book *Switch On Your Brain*, she has a picture of what a healthy memory looks like compared with unhealthy memory.[11] Moreover, the buildup of toxic brain cells sends negative electrical impulses to the rest of the body, creating stress and compromising the immune system.

One of the ways that the brain communicates with the rest of the body is through our blood. As we explained in our earlier book *Juicing, Fasting, and Detoxing for Life*:

> White blood cells have receptor sites for neuropeptides, and when our thoughts are negative, the messengers' (neuropeptides) communication can disrupt the health of our immune cells. Negative thoughts and emotions have been found to decrease T cell production and activity and to release stress hormones. Some neuropeptides can even trigger cancer cells to metastasize. Conversely, others help keep our body healthy.
>
> Chemicals produced by toxic emotions lodge in our muscles and we can experience neck and back pain or pain in other parts of our body. We can experience weakness or intestinal disturbances such as poor digestion, constipation, or diarrhea. The effects of negative emotions are also stored in the liver and kidneys and can disrupt their function and block proper pancreatic function. Unhealthy emotions can also cause cognitive inhibition, affecting our ability to comprehend, think, and make rational decisions. And traumatic memories may trigger allergic reactions. The list could go on and on, but the point to remember is that negative emotions are disruptive to the body, produce toxicity, and can be devastating to our health.[12]

Fortunately, you don't have to be a scientist to tell if a thought, memory, or pattern of thinking is toxic or not. If the thought takes away your joy, if it leads to stress, if it apprehends your peace of mind, or if it makes it harder for you to forgive someone, then the thought is probably toxic.

Examples of toxic thinking would be some of the defense and survival mechanisms I mentioned at the beginning of the previous chapter.

When we try to survive in a state of separateness from our Creator, we activate the reptilian part of the brain and live day to day in an orientation of fight or flight, which is a stress response.

Some further examples of toxic thinking were given in an excellent article that was published by the Taylor Study Method, titled "How Peace of Mind Is a Skill That Can Be Developed With Practice." In the article Robin Phillips describes the brain as "the theater of a constant tug-of-war between the positive and the negative side of us."[13] Phillips continues:

> The more our thought-life empowers the negative side in this tug-of-war the more we will be weighed down and actually make our suffering worse. The tug-of-war between the negative and the positive ultimately determines whether our life will be filled with joy, gratitude, and a sense of hopeful expectancy about the future, or whether our life will be weighed down by grumbling, stress, and a sense of anxiety about the future.[14]

Imagine you know someone whose boyfriend is always tearing her down and continually telling her that she's stupid, that she's unable to cope, that nobody likes her, and that she isn't pretty enough. What would you say to your friend? Obviously you would tell her that she should break up with her negative boyfriend or at least tell him she will not see him any longer if he continues such behavior. Even though that is the advice you would give someone else, when it comes to yourself, do you pay attention to the incessant negative monologue about yourself that is just as bad? The monologue of negativity isn't coming from another person but from your own brain. But instead of "breaking up" with your negative brain, you pay attention to it. If you think I'm exaggerating, just ask yourself the following questions:

+ Does your brain amplify your negative traits while minimizing what is good about you?[15]

+ Do you spend more time thinking about what is wrong in your life than what is positive?[16]

+ Does your mind make hardships worse by dwelling on them over and over again?[17]

+ Do you suffer unnecessarily from imagining future scenarios that may never transpire?[18]

+ Do you allow your brain to fall victim to common thinking errors, such as all-or-nothing thinking, overgeneralizing, catastrophizing, and mind-reading?[19]

+ When challenges arise in your life, does your mind send you defeatist messages, or do you analyze strategies to help you rise above the situation?[20]

+ Do you criticize yourself? Do you think thoughts that say you are not good enough, smart enough, talented enough, good-looking enough, or capable enough?

If you're reading those questions and thinking, "Yes, that's me," don't despair. Both the Bible and modern science show that you don't need to stay in a disordered state of mind. Because the brain is a living organism, it is constantly changing based on how we use it (a phenomenon known as *neuroplasticity*).[21] That means you can start today to retrain your brain by letting go of all negativity. You can form new, positive neuropathways in your brain that lead to peace, joy, and health.

The Power of a Thought

"In a study of the link between emotions and DNA, researchers found that strong emotions alter the shape of one's DNA. Powerful feelings of love were found to unwind, or relax, human DNA strands, whereas high negative emotions, such as frustration, were found to tighten the DNA coils. Furthermore, the study revealed that these effects on one's DNA could be simulated by projecting certain emotional states on one's body. We truly can affect our body's makeup with our thoughts!"[22]

YOU CAN CONTROL YOUR BRAIN AND EMOTIONS

We generally don't have any problem recognizing that many of the problems we face in our bodies are things we can control through healthy choices. For example, if someone has a problem with weight management or low energy, these are problems that can usually be addressed through healthy choices such as exercise, good nutrition, nutritional supplements, juicing, fasting, and detoxing.

When it comes to the brain, however, we often don't appreciate that our thought lives can also be controlled by proper choices. For example, we often assume that our brain controls us and that we are a passive victim of toxic thinking, including painful memories, useless rumination, and ongoing stress about the future. Because we don't understand the power God has given us to control our minds, we often respond to mental stimuli by taking up each thought and entertaining it before another thought takes its place.

"I Think; Therefore, I Am"

Seventeenth-century Europe was a time of great uncertainty. Political turmoil, philosophical and religious innovations, and a series of deadly wars had left Europeans with few verities of which they could still be certain. It was in this climate of uncertainty that the French philosopher and mathematician René Descartes (1596–1650) sought to find a new method for achieving certainty—the perfect method that everyone could agree upon, despite any other differences that might divide them.

In his classic work *Discourse on Method* Descartes proposed that the starting point for the method must be to block out all stimuli from the material world. Mind and matter must be completely separated. Only by first disengaging himself from the stuff of the physical world could Descartes be confident that his mind was unencumbered. Through a process of pure reason Descartes eventually deduced his own existence with his famous *Cogito ergo sum* ("I think; therefore, I am").

Bit by bit he deduced the legitimacy of the physical world and found a place for it within his rationalistic system. Crucially, however, the process he started out with—separating the world of matter from the world of mind—continued to taint his view of the world, which was dominated by what historian Richard Popkin termed a "metaphysical distinction between mind and matter."[23] Philosophers following in the wake of Descartes continued to be tinctured by his philosophy, which came to be known as

"Cartesian dualism." Central to this philosophy was the notion that although mind and body interact, they are totally distinct substances.

Many of us unconsciously assume some form of Cartesian dualism, whereby we view the mind and the body as completely separate entities. Accordingly we often underestimate the extent to which our thought lives affect our bodies. We similarly fail to appreciate the extent to which the brain is a physical organ that we can control just as much as we can control our feet or our hands. Failure to think of the brain as belonging to the same category as the body means that we often treat ourselves as victims of toxic thinking instead of recognizing that we can take control of our brains just as we can control other aspects of our bodies. In fact, research published by the Association for Psychological Science in its journal *Psychological Science* found that perceiving the mind and the body as totally distinct makes a real difference in how we live our lives.[24] "The more people perceive their minds and bodies to be distinct entities, the less likely they will be to engage in behaviors that protect their bodies. Bodies are ultimately viewed as a disposable vessel that helps the mind interact with the physical world."[25]

The same thing happens with our emotions. Often when we feel an emotion such as anger, we think the emotion controls us. In fact, we often talk about emotions as if they *are* us. (For example, we say things such as "I am angry.") Accordingly we think of ourselves as being victims of emotions.

The first step to letting go of toxic emotions or thoughts is recognizing that they are separate from us. Put simply, you are not your thoughts or emotions. Rather, toxic thoughts and feelings are things outside yourself, such as airplanes in the sky, that you can either allow to land in the runway of your heart and mind or reject and watch them fly away.

This type of strenuous control over toxic thoughts and feelings is easier during times of fasting. During a fast the brain slows down, thus making it easier for us to exercise censorship over our thinking. But the functions of the brain are also more enhanced, more controlled, and more at our disposal during times of fasting. This has emerged in a number of different studies. A group of students at the University of Chicago was asked to live for an entire week without food while keeping a regular routine: "Their mental alertness was so much greater during that period that their progress in their school work was cited as remarkable. Several repetitions of this experiment, always with the same results, proved that this was not exceptional."[26] During a fast you can channel this new mental alertness into observing toxic thoughts when they arise and letting them go without taking them up.

Exercising censorship over your thinking doesn't mean just gritting your teeth and saying, "I will not think this negative thought." A person can repeat, "I am not feeling stress" all day long, but that won't make it true. What we need to do is actively replace toxic thinking with the truth. This involves addressing the lies that are behind toxic thinking.

The main lie is that we can survive separate from God. Consider that when we worry about the future, when we ruminate over the past, when we try to grasp a lot of material things for ourselves, or when we chase after the pleasures of life, we are doing exactly as Adam and Eve did when they hid from God: we are acting as if we are separate from the source of life. By contrast, when we focus on what is noble, right, pure, lovely, and admirable (Phil. 4:8), we are connecting with our Creator and beginning to take the journey toward health and wholeness.

BRAIN SCIENCE: HOW TO REWIRE YOUR BRAIN

Toxic thinking may seem like no big deal, but if we engage in toxic thinking long enough, it will actually change how we view ourselves, our loved ones, and the world around us. As psychologist and author Rick Hanson explains:

> Moment to moment, the flows of thoughts and feelings, sensations and desires, and conscious and unconscious processes sculpt your nervous system like water gradually carving furrows and eventually gullies on a hillside. Your brain is continually changing its structure. The only question is: Is it for better or worse?... Attention is like a combination spotlight and vacuum cleaner: it illuminates what it rests upon and then sucks it into your brain—and your self.[27]

The solution is simple: start paying attention to what you're paying attention to. Although this is simple, it's also incredibly difficult. You see, most of us have become so used to following the prompts of our toxic brain that we don't even realize we're doing it anymore. Periods of fasting are the perfect time to begin watching our toxic mental habits and begin forming new ones.

As you take a step back from needing to constantly satisfy the demands of your body by eating throughout the day, you have a chance to also step back from having to constantly meet the demands of your brain. As you discipline your body, you will find it easier to begin disciplining your mind and emotions.

As thoughts arise in your brain, ask yourself, "If I allow this thought to have airtime in my brain, will it help my well-being? Will this draw me closer to my Creator? Will this thought help me grow in gratitude, compassion, forgiveness, and love?" If the answer is no, then let the thought go. As you let go of unhealthy thoughts, sometimes the thoughts will leave, but sometimes they'll stick around. If the unwanted thoughts stick around, that's OK. The important thing is that you are not going to encourage unhealthy thoughts.

In his article "The Most Important 10 Minutes of Your Life" Robin Phillips references an illustration given by Chade-Meng Tan in the book *Search Inside Yourself*, saying, "He compares unwanted thoughts to monsters. If your house happens to get overrun by monsters, you have three choices. Either you can feed the monsters, in which case they will stick around. Or you can fight the monsters, in which case you may get clobbered and defeated with the result that the monsters become stronger. Or you can do your best to simply ignore the monsters. If you choose to ignore the monsters, maybe they will go away or maybe they won't, but even if they stick around, you will have learned to treat them with the contempt they deserve and they will have lost their hold over you."[28] Practice this long enough, and you will actually rewire the neurocircuitry of your brain.

Science supports the approach I am urging. Neuroscientist Dr. Caroline Leaf has been involved in helping victims of traumatic brain injury to recover. She has been able to apply the same principles in helping people whose thought lives had been taken over by stressful patterns of thinking. Her discoveries can benefit us all. In her book *Switch On Your Brain* Dr. Leaf shares about what she learned:

> I was struck by how my patients, using the therapeutic techniques I was developing from my research, belied the negative picture conventional science presented of the human brain at that time. These results confirmed that the brain, far from being fixed in toxicity, can change even in the most challenging neurological situations.
>
> I was in awe of what each patient displayed in terms of what you can do when you set your mind to it. Each new scientific study in this direction confirmed what I knew intuitively to be true: We are not victims of our biology or circumstances. How we react to the events and circumstances of life can have an enormous impact on our mental and even physical health.
>
> As we think, we change the physical nature of our brain. As we consciously direct our thinking, we can wire out toxic patterns of thinking and replace them with healthy thoughts. New thought networks grow. We increase our intelligence and bring healing to our brains, minds, and physical bodies.[29]

Later on in the same book Dr. Leaf explains what it looks like in practice to rewire toxic patterns of thinking:

> Research dating back to the 1970s shows that capturing our thoughts in a disciplined way rather than letting them chaotically run rampant can bring about impressive changes in how we feel and think. This change is evidenced in cognitive, emotional functioning as well as at the neural level....
>
> When you objectively observe your own thinking with the view to capturing rogue thoughts, you in effect direct your attention to stop the negative impact and rewire healthy new circuits into your brain....
>
> When you make a conscious decision to focus and direct your attention correctly, you change physical matter—your brain and your body change in a healthy way. Purposefully catching your thoughts can control the brain's sensory processing, the brain's rewiring, the neurotransmitters, the genetic expression, and

cellular activity in a positive or negative direction....Not catching
those thoughts will lead to a potential spiral into confusion and
varying levels of mental despair.[30]

MASTERING THE SOUL: LETTING GO OF TOXIC EMOTIONS

It was early summer but already hot for the season. I had spent the first
part of the morning sitting on my deck overlooking Lake Coeur d'Alene,
praying about our upcoming wellness retreat. I reflected on how many
people come to our retreats to detoxify their bodies through a juice fast.
When they leave five days later, many have also experienced the life-
changing blessing of being able to detoxify their hearts and souls from
toxic emotions.

One of the highlights of our retreats is my having the opportunity to
explain heart-rate variability. During times of stress and negative emotions the rhythm of the heart is disordered, a state cardiologists call *inco-
herence*. During these times, "the pattern of neural signals traveling from
the heart to the brain" is disordered, leading to a decrease in the higher
cognitive functions (attention, perception, memory, emotional intelligence,
problem-solving skills, and so forth).[31] This decrease in proper cognition
leaves people without the inner resources for dealing with stress, which, in
turn, reinforces the negative emotions underlying the heart's disordered
pattern of beating. This is the fight-or-flight condition in which so many
people spend their entire lives without even realizing it.

By contrast, when our emotional life is characterized by feelings of gratitude, compassion, love, appreciation, and peace, the rhythm of the heart
exists in a state of *coherence*. This is not a state of relaxation but a state of
well-being that we often feel when we're in the presence of someone who
radiates peace, compassion, and inner warmth to us. Having a coherent
heart rate initiates a positive web of reciprocities in the mind and body,
resulting in increased mental, emotional, and physical fitness.

That Heart Rate Matters

"Most of us have been taught in school that the heart is constantly responding to 'orders' sent by the brain in the form of neural signals. However, it is not as commonly known that the heart actually sends more signals to the brain than the brain sends to the heart! Moreover, these heart signals have a significant effect on brain function—influencing emotional processing as well as higher cognitive faculties such as attention, perception, memory, and problem-solving. In other words, not only does the heart respond to the brain, but the brain continuously responds to the heart. . . .

"During stress and negative emotions, when the heart rhythm pattern is erratic and disordered, the corresponding pattern of neural signals traveling from the heart to the brain inhibits higher cognitive functions. This limits our ability to think clearly, remember, learn, reason, and make effective decisions. (This helps explain why we may often act impulsively and unwisely when we're under stress.) The heart's input to the brain during stressful or negative emotions also has a profound effect on the brain's emotional processes—actually serving to reinforce the emotional experience of stress.

"In contrast, the more ordered and stable pattern of the heart's input to the brain during positive emotional states has the opposite effect—it facilitates cognitive function and reinforces positive feelings and emotional stability. This means that learning to generate increased heart rhythm coherence, by sustaining positive emotions, not only benefits the entire body, but also profoundly affects how we perceive, think, feel, and perform. . . .

"Research has also shown that the heart is a key component of the emotional system. Scientists now understand that the heart not only responds to emotion, but that the signals generated by its rhythmic activity actually play a major part in determining the quality of our emotional experience from moment to moment."[32]

That morning as I sat on my deck, I was thinking about how best to present some of the new research from neurocardiologists on the link between emotion and heart health. I was just getting ready to go in and see if Cherie needed anything when there was a knock on our door.

"Who could that be?" I thought. Then I remembered that a man, whom I'll call Jim, had made an appointment to come and see me. He wanted to talk about the emWave, an extremely sophisticated device that researchers at HeartMath developed to monitor the rhythm of the heart. Whereas equipment used by doctors will typically tell you how many beats you have over a period of time (i.e., sixty-five beats a minute), as well as blood pressure, the emWave measures the rhythm of the heart. Through a complex process of biofeedback the device can measure second by second whether someone's heart is in a state of coherence (heart-rate variability) or whether the heartbeat is disordered and incoherent. Increasing numbers of people are using the emWave throughout the day to monitor their heart rates to know when they need to apply techniques such as appreciative thinking, deep breathing, and fasting from toxic emotions.

Almost as soon as I let Jim into the house, he came straight to the point. "Can you tell me more about the emWave?" he asked.

"Yes," I replied. "I'll get it out in due course. But first I'd like to learn a little about you and why you're interested in this."

He began explaining a bit about his situation. It turned out that he was weathering a series of personal and professional crises, the stress of which had been affecting his health, including his ability to think properly. He didn't go into a lot of details, but it was clear that the stress of his situation had left him trapped in a cycle of toxic emotions and thoughts. His focus had shifted from living to simply surviving.

Jim didn't want to talk too much about his troubles but to get down to the business of why he had come. "What techniques can I apply to have a healthy heart and not feel stressed all the time?" he asked.

I connected him to the emWave to measure his heart-rate variability. Not surprisingly the biofeedback readings showed that his heart rate wasn't in a state of coherence. I encouraged Jim to take some deep breaths, to visualize the breathing coming in and out of his heart, and to reflect on some things he appreciated. Suddenly the light on the emWave turned green, showing that his heart-rate variability had entered a state of coherence.

Concerned that maybe it was just a coincidence, he said that he was going to think a negative thought and see if it changed the biofeedback readings. Before he even had time to think the negative thought, the light turned red, showing he had lost coherence. He was amazed. Simply anticipating thinking a negative thought is enough to cause a stress response in your body. (For more information on the emWave, see the Resources appendix.)

After a few minutes I asked him to put the device down. I looked deeply at him and then said, "You know, I could spend all day training you in the techniques for achieving heart-rate variability. And that's important. We will talk more about that. But what is even more important is that we address the root cause of your stress. I don't want to simply mask over the problem. In order for you to have a healthy heart, a healthy brain, and a healthy body, we need to get to the bottom of why you so easily feel stress."

"So what is the root cause of my stress?" he asked.

"Let me just say," I responded, "that I have some good news for you and some bad news."

"Let's have the good news first," he replied eagerly.

"The good news is that there is a God. The bad news is that He's not you."

I went on to explain that the stress and anxiety that were dominating his life arose from his attempts to be God. What he was discovering was that he wasn't very good at being God.

"I'm not trying to be God," he replied defensively. "What are you talking about?"

"When we try to be God," I explained, "then our survival depends on ourselves. But when we let go of trying to be God, we stop thinking that everything depends on us. We can let go. This is what it means to fast from toxic thinking and toxic emotions."

I went on to explain that when we try to be our own God, there are three things that happen, all of which create stress. One is that we want to control others. Two, we want other people's praise. Three, we seek to judge other people. A large percentage of our stress arises from these three areas.

I'd like to unpack each of these three areas, one at a time, that I shared with Jim that morning.

Trying to be God: attempting to control

God is in control of everything. When we try to control people and situations in our lives—that is, when we try to do God's job—we find that we aren't very good at it. Somehow, people refuse to let us control them, even when we are trying to influence them for their own good or the good of other people. People fail to see and correct problems that seem obvious to us and that we have tried to point out. Even the people we have authority over and whom we have a responsibility to exercise limited control over often refuse to follow our leads.

Maybe you don't think of yourself as being a control freak. Few people do. But ask yourself the following questions:[33]

+ **Does it bother you when you're not in control?** When we attempt to be in control over things beyond our power of influence, it produces anxiety, stress, and worry.[34]

+ **Does it bother you when things don't go your way?** When things don't go your way and you are troubled by that, ask yourself if you think God isn't doing things the right way in your life.[35]

+ **Do you have trouble asking for help?** Not wanting to ask for help might stem from pride in your own abilities to handle all situations in your life. Do you try to be independent and self-sufficient?[36]

+ **Do you try to change people?** You may have set a standard for how people should be, act, and think. Do you try to get people to conform to your standard?

When we find that we are not able to control people very well, there are two ways we can respond. One is to become stressed out and struggle against our lack of control. This struggle can take the form of trying new ways to exert control and manipulate people. Or it can take the form of anger. Or it can take the form of worry and anxiety as we dwell on the problem. The other alternative is to not struggle at all but to let go of trying to control. We can rejoice in the fact that we don't have the burden of being in control of all things. We can leave God to exercise His omnipotence in the way He knows is best.

Trying to be God: seeking praise

All honor and praise are due to God. He is the One who created you, not yourself. When we seek to receive honor and praise for ourselves—that is, when we try to be God—we find it doesn't work very well. Something always seems to happen to bring us down from our pedestal. Maybe we make a mistake in public. Maybe someone gossips about us or falsely accuses us. Or maybe people simply don't appreciate all the good qualities we think we have.

Ask yourself the following questions:

+ **Do you look for approval or thanks from others?**
  When we look for approval or praise from others, we're
  seeking the praise due to God.[37]

+ **Do you get impatient when people don't do things
  right?** Impatience with others shows that we've judged
  them and they aren't living up to our standards.[38]

+ **Do you try to keep people happy?** Working to keep
  people happy is a form of control. We can never be the
  source of another person's happiness.[39]

When we find that people do not praise us, we again are presented with a choice. We can struggle against this and have stress. Or we can acknowledge that God deserves the praise.

Trying to be God: exercising judgment

There's only one who is truly capable of being judge, and that is God. When we judge others, we're saying we know better than God how people should act, how they should treat us, how they should do things, and how they should respond to life. Ask yourself the following question:

+ **Do I get impatient or irritated when people don't do
  things right?** Impatience indicates that you have a standard that other people are violating.[40]

+ **Do you try to change people?** This indicates that you
  have a standard for people that you want them to live up
  to.

When we try to be our own God, our survival depends on watching out for ourselves. Our minds become hypervigilant to perceived threats, slights, or injustices, resulting in stress. We begin thinking things such as:

+ What is that person thinking about me right now?
  (wanting praise)

+ How can I influence other people in this situation or
  manipulate a situation to get what I want? (wanting to
  control)

+ How can I establish that I am right and he or she is
  wrong? (wanting to judge)

All these toxic patterns of thinking arise from taking up the burden of our own survival, a burden God never intended for us to have. By contrast, when we learn to let go, we can replace toxic thinking with the mind of Christ.

The section that follows will offer step-by-step guidance on this letting-go process.

THE TWENTY-ONE-DAY MENTAL AND EMOTIONAL FAST

As you fast from various foods and drinks, you have the wonderful opportunity to also fast from emotions and thoughts that choke the soul. We have a little game we play with Annie Mae, our eight-year-old schnauzer. It's actually a game with a purpose. If there are birds at the windowsill pecking on the front window and making a mess on the ledge, or if there are wild turkeys in the driveway doing the same, we say, "Get the bad ones!" Annie Mae will run to the front door and bark, sending them on their way. If only we could just bark at the "bad ones" of our souls and they would take flight! But it takes a little more work for us.

In the following section we address six major areas of toxic emotions and provide exercises to help you let go of them. We strongly encourage you to work through all six areas and the related exercises, even if you think you don't have a challenge in a given area. If you approach these exercises with openness, you may be surprised what you discover about yourself.

Within each of the major categories of negative emotions we have included numerous subcategories. For example, you might not express unrighteous anger often (there is a righteous anger), but you might become easily impatient or irritated, both of which are subcategories of anger. You might not have a problem with lust, but you might struggle with envy. Approach this emotional fast with an open mind and heart.

Before getting started, ask yourself the following questions. And if it helps, get out a piece of paper and write a response to each one:

+ What are the main areas of mental and emotional toxicity (negative emotions and thoughts) for me?

+ What effect are toxic thoughts and emotions having on my health and well-being?

+ What would my life and relationships be like if I was freed from toxic emotions and thoughts?

+ Do I believe I can release these toxic emotions and thoughts? Why? Why not?

We suggest you tackle two categories of emotions per week in your twenty-one-day emotional detox fast.

Week 1: anger and apathy

You may not think you have a problem with anger. However, anger is the root of an entire family of toxic emotions such as irritation or frustration. Some of the sub-emotions that spring from the root of anger include:

Aggressive, annoyed, argumentative, defiant, demanding, disgusted, frustrated, furious, hateful, impatient, irritated, jealous, mad, mean, outraged, resentful, retaliatory, spiteful, sullen, vengeful, vicious, and violent

Throughout this week read through that list a few times and circle the emotions that apply to you. This is your week to fast from these emotions. Acknowledge that you are fasting from anger, even if your particular issue relates to one of the subcategories. If you are sullen, impatient, or annoyed, the root is still anger and needs to be addressed.

It's easy to fool ourselves. We may say, "I was only slightly irritated. I wasn't angry." But we have an opportunity to acknowledge the root of the emotion so we can let it go.

Also this week spend time doing some soul-searching about the emotion of apathy. Apathy isn't an emotion we tend to talk about a lot in our culture, but it's at the root of a number of other emotions that can choke our soul. Here are some emotions and thought patterns related to apathy:

Bored, careless, defeated, depressed, discouraged, disillusioned, drained, futile, hopeless, helpless, insensitive, overwhelmed, powerless, resigned, wasted, withdrawn, and worthless

Circle any of those subcategories that apply to you. By identifying the applicable subcategories, you'll be in a position to let go of the primary emotions. For example, if you recognize that you feel defeated or hopeless, this will alert you that you need to let go of the root emotion of apathy. By putting your focus on the primary emotion, you will be able to address the sub-emotions effectively.

This week the focus of your emotional fast is anger and apathy. These are the emotions you will work on letting go of. See the section that follows on the "letting-go process" for more on how to do this.

Week 2: Fear and grief

You may not think you have a problem with either fear or grief. However, we learned in week 1 that there are many root emotions that spawn an entire family of sub-feelings. It's the same with fear and grief.

Some of the sub-emotions that spring from fear include worry and insecurity.

> Anxious, apprehensive, cautious, cowardly, doubtful, foreboding, inhibited, insecure, nervous, panicky, scared, shaky, trapped, and worried

Similarly grief is at the root of a number of toxic feelings, including such emotions as rejection and anguish.

> Abandoned, abused, accused, anguished, ashamed, betrayed, cheated, embarrassed, helpless, hurt, ignored, left out, misunderstood, neglected, rejected, sad, and slighted

During this week spend your days focusing on fear and grief and their sub-categories. Circle the subcategories that apply to you, and ask yourself the crucial questions from the "Letting-Go" section.

Remember that I said before there are no right or wrong answers to these questions, provided you are being honest. This is especially true when dealing with grief. If you have suffered severe grief or trauma—for example, if you have lost a loved one, experienced divorce, or endured a tragedy—it is healthy to let yourself experience the grieving process. You might say, "Yes, I can let this go, but I'm not ready yet." You may be able to let it go in stages. Again, that's OK. But eventually you will reach a point where you can say, "Now I'm ready to *completely* let this go and move on with my life."

Week 3: lust and pride

Although lust and pride are things that most humans struggle with, they are also the two areas we are least likely to admit to struggling with. Again, it's helpful to review the subcategories:

> **Lust:** This is the emotion that yells, "I want!" Offshoot emotions include anticipation, craving, demanding, desiring, feeling devious, driven, envious, frustrated, greedy, manipulating, obsessive, ruthless, selfish, and wicked.

Pride: The subcategories of pride include emotions such as feeling aloof, arrogant, boastful, clever, contemptuous, cool, critical, judgmental, righteous, rigid, self-satisfied, selfish, snobbish, spoiled, superior, unforgiving, and vain.

This week, spend some time looking over these sub-emotions and circling the ones you're experiencing. All the subcategories point to the main emotions of pride or lust. Again, they back up to the core emotion. For example, if you are driven to gratify your desires, such as finding joy and comfort by eating sweets, gaining excitement by shopping a lot, or feeding your ego with achievement, you may not think that this is as bad as lust, yet it's important to recognize that the root emotion is indeed lust.

The letting-go process (also called the Sedona Method)

As you let go of toxic emotions, work through the following steps. Also use these steps to let go of toxic thinking. Whenever a thought enters your mind that is critical, judgmental, hurtful, or that steals your peace, let it go. Here's the process:[41]

Focus

Identify the problem or set of problems in your life that lead to certain feelings. Find the core emotion that is at the root of what you are feeling. For example, the core emotion behind spitefulness is anger, while the core emotion behind envy is lust. These are toxic emotions that you will be greatly served by letting go of.

Feel

Zero in on how you feel. We're often afraid to admit how we're really feeling, with the result that we suppress our emotions. However, even when we suppress toxic emotions, they're still there, affecting our spiritual and physical health.

In her insightful book *Feelings Buried Alive Never Die* Karol Truman says:

> Incorrect or not, that perception [feeling/emotion] has been stored in our cells—in our DNA—covering over the memory…[has]

been carried with us throughout our years, often creating enormous physical, emotional, or mental pain in some area of our life. Our mind had to draw some conclusion for the discomfort (pain) we felt at the time the core incident occurred. Consequently, whatever data was available in our subconscious from previous experiences for us to reference, determined the belief we established, whether correct or incorrect.[42]

A past stored emotion can get triggered by current events. That is why Cherie said the emotional pain of the burglar attack connected with all the pain from her past felt like an emotional tsunami. She had to get to core emotions to let go of it all.

Now, go to the week you are in for your twenty-one-day emotional detox program to identify the two major feelings that come up in that week. For example, if you are in week 1, identify all feelings that are associated with anger and apathy. When appropriate—such as with emotions of anger, fear, or grief—allow your body to experience the full force of the emotion. Perhaps you will cry or shake. That's OK.

Ask yourself, "Could I let it go?"

A key aspect to emotional maturity is being able to distinguish between our emotions and our true selves. One of the ways we can do this is by asking the simple question, "Could I let this feeling go?" Perhaps you will answer yes, perhaps no, perhaps maybe one day. It's important to realize that there are no wrong answers—just be honest.

Ask yourself, "Would I let it go?"

Maybe you recognized that you *could* let go of a toxic emotion, but you're not yet ready to actually let it go. For example, if you're feeling deep grief at a loss or feeling anger or rage at a wrong that was committed against you or a loved one and you're not yet ready to let go of the feeling, that's OK. For this exercise to work, you have to be honest with yourself. Again, answer honestly, whether it's yes, no, or maybe.

When?

It could be now, tomorrow, next month, or never. Whatever your answer is, that's OK. Just keep repeating this exercise until such a time as your answer is, "Now I'm ready to be released from this toxic feeling."

Letting go

As you continue this process, there will be a time when you can answer each of the questions in a way that brings about a release. As you release the emotions, you may feel a wave of relief throughout your body. You may break into uncontrollable tears or maybe even laughter. Or you may simply experience a warmth in your heart or a calm sense in your soul and the freedom of no longer being bound by the toxic emotion. Whichever way your body reacts, that's OK.

For many people this process of letting go is a one-time thing, and the toxic emotion never returns again. Others have to repeat the process of letting go regularly, sometimes every day. The most important thing is not to give up. If it takes a long period of time to be fully released from the toxic emotion, be patient with yourself. Just keep letting go.

In summary, each time you experience the toxic feelings for the week you're in, 1) identify the feeling, 2) let yourself feel the feeling, and 3) ask the following questions:

- Could I let it go?
- Would I let it go?
- When?

Keep up this process until you experience release.

Enjoying the Freedom

Congratulations! You've made it to the end of your twenty-one-day mental and emotional fast. Take some time to reflect over the last three weeks. If you're the sort of person who enjoys journaling, write down some answers to the following questions:

+ How did you feel before beginning the emotional/mental fast?

+ How do you feel now that you have finished?

+ What did you learn about yourself in the process?

+ What was the most important lesson you learned during this time?

+ How will this make a difference as you move forward in ordinary life?

As normal life takes over, be prepared to experience some setbacks. If you find yourself slipping back to your old toxic patterns of thinking and feeling, don't be discouraged. Remember that inner healing isn't a one-time process but an ongoing journey. Again, for some people, the process of letting go is experienced in a dramatic one-time event, but more often it is something we have to keep doing every day.

As you experience the various sub-emotions associated with anger, apathy, fear, grief, lust, or pride, simply turn to God and let go. If you have to do this a hundred times in one day, that's OK. Just keep letting go.

We will always have emotions and thoughts that are not life-giving that try to sneak into our souls. Keep at the work of letting go. Be aware of what you think and feel, just as you are aware of what you eat and drink. The main thing is to remain open to listening to your heart, which is where God speaks to us. Enjoy the freedom that only letting go can bring.

RESOURCES

NEWSLETTER

Sign up for Cherie's Juicy Tips Newsletter. Get a free recipe and 10 percent off your first order for signing up; also get recipes and healthy tips twice a week from America's most trusted nutritionist. Go to www .juiceladyinfo.com.

CHERIE'S WEBSITES

For information on juicing and weight loss, go to:

+ www.juiceladyinfo.com
+ www.juiceladycherie.com
+ www.cheriecalbom.com

CHERIE'S PROGRAMS

The Juice Lady's Health and Wellness Juice & Raw Foods Cleanse Retreats

I invite you to join us for a week that can change your life! Our retreats offer gourmet, organic raw foods with a three-day juice fast midweek. We present interesting, informative classes in a beautiful, peaceful setting where you can experience healing and restoration of body and soul.

For more information and dates for the retreats, visit http://www .juiceladycherie.com/Juice/juice-raw-food-retreat or call 866-843-8935.

The Thirty-Day Sugar Detox

This four-week e-course with a lesson each week helps you embrace your own healthy, sugarless lifestyle that you can stick with for life. Learn how to overcome your sweet tooth. Learn to make healthy desserts that don't mess up your blood sugar. You'll also get private Facebook coaching and a teleconference call each week with Cherie.

For more information, go to http://www.juiceladycherie.com/Juice /healthy-and-fit-for-life or call 866-843-8935.

The Juice Lady's 30-Day Detox Challenge

This is a four-week e-course designed to help your body get rid of toxins, contaminants, waste, and heavy metals that can accumulate in joints, organs, tissues, cells, the lymphatic system, and the bloodstream. It can energize your entire body. You'll get an e-lesson each week, private Facebook coaching with Cherie, and a teleconference call each week during which you can ask questions.

For more information, go to http://www.juiceladycherie.com /Juice/30-day-detox or call 866-843-8935.

The Mini-Cleanse—seven-day colon cleanse

For more information, go to http://www.juiceladycherie.com.

The 5-Day Juice Fast

This is a five-day juice fast with a downloadable lesson for each day, private Facebook coaching, and a teleconference call with Cherie. For more information or to register, go to www.juiceladyinfo.com.

Nutrition counseling

To schedule a nutrition consultation with the Juice Lady's team, visit http://www.juiceladycherie.com/Juice/nutritional-counseling or call 866-843-8935.

Scheduling Cherie Calbom to speak

To schedule Cherie Calbom to speak for your organization, call 866-843-8935.

Books by Cherie and John Calbom

These books can be ordered at any of the websites above or by calling 866-843-8935.

* Cherie Calbom, *The Juice Lady's Remedies for Diabetes* (Siloam)

* Cherie Calbom, *Sugar Knockout* (Siloam)

* Cherie Calbom and Abby Fammartino, *The Juice Lady's Anti-Inflammation Diet* (Siloam)

* Cherie Calbom, *The Juice Lady's Big Book of Juices and Green Smoothies* (Siloam)

* Cherie Calbom, *The Juice Lady's Remedies for Asthma and Allergies* (Siloam)

* Cherie Calbom, *The Juice Lady's Remedies for Stress and Adrenal Fatigue* (Siloam)

* Cherie Calbom, *The Juice Lady's Weekend Weight-Loss Diet* (Siloam)

* Cherie Calbom, *The Juice Lady's Living Foods Revolution* (Siloam)

* Cherie Calbom, *The Juice Lady's Turbo Diet* (Siloam)

* Cherie Calbom, *The Juice Lady's Guide to Juicing for Health* (Avery)

* Cherie Calbom and John Calbom, *Juicing, Fasting, and Detoxing for Life* (Wellness Central)

* Cherie Calbom, *The Wrinkle Cleanse* (Avery)

* Cherie Calbom and John Calbom, *The Coconut Diet* (Wellness Central)

* Cherie Calbom, John Calbom, and Michael Mahaffey, *The Complete Cancer Cleanse* (Thomas Nelson)

* Cherie Calbom, *The Ultimate Smoothie Book* (Wellness Central)

Juicers

To find out about the best juicers recommended by Cherie, call 866-843-8935 or visit www.juiceladyinfo.com.

Dehydrators

To find out about the best dehydrators recommended by Cherie, call 866-843-8935 or visit www.juiceladyinfo.com.

Veggie powders and supplements

To purchase or get information on Garden's Best Superfood Powder, Wheatgrass Juice Powder, and Bone Broth Powder, go to www. juiceladyinfo.com or call 866-843-8935. These powders are ideal for when you travel or while fasting. You can mix them in your juice to add nutritional benefits or use them when you can't get juice.

Internal cleansing kits

The complete and comprehensive internal cleansing kit contains eighteen items for a twenty-one-day cleanse program. You will receive a free colon cleanse kit, along with Liver-Gallbladder Rejuvenator, Friendly Bacteria Replenisher, Parasite Cleanser, Lung Rejuvenator, Kidney and Bladder Rejuvenator, Blood and Skin Rejuvenator, and Lymph Rejuvenator. See one of the websites listed for more information.

You may order the cleansing products and get the 10 percent discount by calling 866-843-8935.

Berry Breeze

Keep your produce fresher longer and your fridge smelling fresh too. It can save you up to $2,200 a year from lost produce. Go to www.juice ladycherie.com.

EmWave2

The EmWave2 is a cardio biofeedback device that provides "heart rhythm feedback and training in real time to help you shift to a positive emotional state in a moment. As a hand held device, you can use it at anytime. Then, connect it to your computer for new sessions, games and access to the HeartCloud."[1] It will help you transform your response to stress and quickly rebalance your mind, body, and emotions. You'll be able to think more clearly, become more intuitive, and make better decisions. And you'll improve your health, resilience, and well-being.

Cleanse products

For more information on the cleanse kits and Digestive Stimulator or Colon Max, see www.juiceladyinfo.com.

Colon Cleanse Kit

This contains Toxin Absorber—fiber and bentonite clay—and the herbal supplement Digestive Stimulator.

Parasite Cleanse Kit

This contains herbs to help you get rid of parasites.

Find out more about the cleanse kits at www.juiceladycherie.com.

NOTES

CHAPTER 1—THE BENEFITS OF FASTING

1. *Los Angeles Times*, "The Fasting Diet…," *Chicago Tribune*, February 7, 2009, accessed September 2, 2016, http://articles.chicagotribune.com/2009-02-07/news /0902060398_1_fasting-calorie-american-dietetic-association.
2. "History of Fasting," All About Fasting, accessed September 2, 2016, http://www .allaboutfasting.com/history-of-fasting.html.
3. Jason Fung, "Fasting—A History Part 1," Intensive Dietary Management, accessed September 2, 2016, https://intensivedietarymanagement.com/fasting-a -history-part-i/.
4. Ibid.
5. Ibid.
6. "History of Fasting."
7. Ibid.
8. Fung, "Fasting—A History Part 1."
9. Emma Young, "Deprive Yourself: The Real Benefits of Fasting," *New Scientist*, November 14, 2012, accessed September 2, 2016, https://www.newscientist.com /article/mg21628912-400-deprive-yourself-the-real-benefits-of-fasting/.
10. Anahad O'Connor, "Fasting Diets Are Gaining Acceptance," *Well* (blog), *New York Times*, March 7, 2016, accessed September 2, 2016, http://well.blogs.nytimes .com/2016/03/07/intermittent-fasting-diets-are-gaining-acceptance/?_r=1.
11. Ibid.
12. Ibid.
13. Carol Torgan, "Health Effects of a Diet That Mimics Fasting," National Institutes of Health, July 13, 2015, accessed September 2, 2016, https://www.nih.gov/news -events/nih-research-matters/health-effects-diet-mimics-fasting.
14. Ibid.
15. Ibid.
16. *Merriam-Webster Online*, s.v. "fast," accessed September 2, 2016, http://www .merriam-webster.com/dictionary/fasting.
17. Jennifer Eivaz, "Fasting Can Be a Game Changer for This," *Charisma News*, April 17, 2016, accessed September 2, 2016, http://www.charismanews.com/opinion /56543-fasting-can-be-a-game-changer-for-this.
18. "Water Fasting," All About Fasting, accessed September 2, 2016, http://www.all aboutfasting.com/water-fasting.html.
19. Linda Carney, "Using Diet to Cut Off Blood Supply to Tumors," DrCarney.com, June 6, 2014, accessed September 2, 2016, http://www.drcarney.com/blog/entry /using-diet-to-cut-off-blood-supply-to-tumors.
20. Peter Seewald, ed., *Wisdom From the Monastery: A Program of Spiritual Healing* (Old Saybrook, CT: Konecky & Konecky, 2004), 30.
21. Emma Young, "Fasting May Protect Against Disease; Some Say It May Even Be Good for the Brain," *Washington Post*, December 31, 2012, accessed September 2, 2016, https://www.washingtonpost.com/national/health-science/fasting-may

-protect-against-disease-some-say-it-may-even-be-good-for-the-brain
/2012/12/24/6e521ee8-3588-11e2-bb9b-288a310849ee_story.html.

22. Ibid.

23. Ibid.

24. Herbert Shelton, "How Diseases Are Cured," DrBass.com, accessed September 2, 2016, http://www.drbass.com/disease-cure.html.

25. Alan Goldhamer, "The Benefits of Fasting," T. Colin Campbell Center for Nutritional Studies, November 1, 1997, accessed September 2, 2016, http://nutrition studies.org/benefits-fasting/.

26. J. Kjeldsen-Kragh et al., "Controlled Trial of Fasting and One-Year Vegetarian Diet in Rheumatoid Arthritis," *Lancet* 338 (October 12, 1991): 899–902; H. Muller, F. W. de Toledo, and K. L. Resch, "Fasting Followed by Vegetarian Diet in Patients With Rheumatoid Arthritis: A Systematic Review," *Scandinavian Journal of Rheumatology* 30, no. 1 (2001): 1–10; J. Palmblad, I. Hafström, and B. Ringertz, "Antirheumatic Effects of Fasting," *Rheumatic Diseases Clinics of North America* 17, no. 2 (May 1991): 351–362.

27. Seewald, ed., *Wisdom From the Monastery*, 31.

28. David Jockers, "Intermittent Fasting SuperCharges Your Brain," Primal Docs, accessed September 2, 2016, http://primaldocs.com/members-blog/intermittent -fasting-supercharges-your-brain/.

29. Ibid.

30. Ibid.

31. Ibid.

32. Seewald, ed., *Wisdom From the Monastery*, 18.

33. Allan Cott, *Fasting: The Ultimate Diet* (n.p.: Hastings House, 1996), as quoted in "Using Fasting for Weight Loss," All About Fasting, accessed September 2, 2016, http://www.allaboutfasting.com/fasting-for-weight-loss.html.

34. G. Vistoli et al., "Advanced Glycoxidation and Lipoxidation End Products (AGEs and ALEs): An Overview of Their Mechanisms of Formation," *Free Radical Research* 47, suppl. 1 (August 2013): 3–27.

35. Alison Goldin et al., "Advanced Glycation End Products," *Circulation* 114, issue 6 (August 8, 2006).

36. University of Southern California, "Diet That Mimics Fasting Appears to Slow Aging," Science Daily, June 18, 2015, accessed September 2, 2016, https://www .sciencedaily.com/releases/2015/06/150618134408.htm.

37. Ibid.

38. Ibid.

39. Rafael De Cabo et al., "The Search for Anti-Aging Interventions: From Elixirs to Fasting Regimens," *Cell* 157, no. 7 (June 19, 2014): 1515–1526.

40. Carolyn H. Dickerson, "The Benefits of Juicing to Reverse Aging Naturally," LookGreat-LoseWeight-SaveMoney.com, accessed September 2, 2016, http:// www.lookgreat-loseweight-savemoney.com/benefits-of-juicing.html.

41. Hans Diehl, "The Story of Ann Wigmore," EnCognitive.com, accessed September 2, 2016, http://www.encognitive.com/node/4200.

42. Fung, "Fasting—A History Part 1."

43. Jockers, "Intermittent Fasting SuperCharges Your Brain."

44. National Institute on Aging, "Can We Prevent Aging?," February 2012, updated July 29, 2016, accessed September 2, 2016, https://www.nia.nih.gov/health /publication/can-we-prevent-aging.

45. Stephanie Bair, "Intermittent Fasting: Try This at Home for Brain Health," *Law and Biosciences Blog*, January 9, 2015, accessed September 2, 2016, https://law .stanford.edu/2015/01/09/lawandbiosciences-2015-01-09-intermittent-fasting-try -this-at-home-for-brain-health/.

46. Arjun Walia, "Neuroscientist Shows What Fasting Does to Your Brain and Why Big Pharma Won't Study It," Collective-Evolution.com, December 11, 2015, accessed September 2, 2016, http://www.collective-evolution.com/2015/12/11 /neuroscientist-shows-what-fasting-does-to-your-brain-why-big-pharma-wont- study-it/).

47. Ibid.

48. Ibid.

49. Suzanne Wu, "Fasting Triggers Stem Cell Regeneration of Damaged, Old Immune System," *USC News*, June 5, 2014, accessed September 2, 2016, https:// news.usc.edu/63669/fasting-triggers-stem-cell-regeneration-of-damaged-old -immune-system/.

50. Walia, "Neuroscientist Shows What Fasting Does to Your Brain and Why Big Pharma Won't Study It."

CHAPTER 2—THE DIFFERENT FASTING DIETS

1. Michael F. Picco, "Digestion: How Long Does It Take?," Mayo Clinic, accessed September 6, 2016, http://www.mayoclinic.org/digestive-system/expert-answers /faq-20058340.

2. L. Bondolfi et al., "Impact of Age and Caloric Restriction on Neurogenesis in the Dentate Gyrus of C57BL/6 Mice," *Neurobiology of Aging* 25, no. 3 (March 2004): 333–340, as referenced in "11 Ways to Grow New Brain Cells and Stimulate Neurogenesis," *Mental Health Daily* (blog), accessed September 6, 2016, http:// mentalhealthdaily.com/2013/03/05/11-ways-to-grow-new-brain-cells-and -stimulate-neurogenesis/.

3. Environmental Working Group, "Body Burden: The Pollution in Newborns," July 14, 2005, accessed September 6, 2016, http://www.ewg.org/research/body -burden-pollution-newborns.

4. Cynthia Foster, "The Healing Power of Juicing," accessed September 6, 2016, http://www.drfostersessentials.com/store/juicing.php.

5. Food Babe, "Don't Fall Victim to These Tricky Food Labels," November 10, 2013, accessed September 6, 2016, http://foodbabe.com/2013/11/10/juice-labels/.

6. *Easton's Bible Dictionary*, s.v. "pulse," accessed September 6, 2016, http://www .biblestudytools.com/dictionary/pulse/.

7. United States Department of Agriculture, "All About the Fruit Group," updated July 26, 2016, accessed September 6, 2016, http://www.choosemyplate.gov /fruit#sthash.6hZKKsOf.dpuf.

8. United States Department of Agriculture, "All About the Vegetable Group," updated July 26, 2016, accessed September 6, 2016, http://www.choosemyplate .gov/vegetables#sthash.OjPiXtxp.dpuf.

9. United States Department of Agriculture, "All About the Grains Group," updated July 26, 2016, accessed September 6, 2016, http://www.choosemyplate.gov /grains#sthash.TLDDyAYz.dpuf.

10. United States Department of Agriculture, "All About the Protein Foods Group," updated July 29, 2016, accessed September 6, 2016, https://www.choosemyplate .gov/protein-foods.

11. Josh Axe, "Bone Broth Benefits for Digestion, Arthritis, and Cellulite," DrAxe. com, accessed September 6, 2016, http://draxe.com/the-healing-power-of-bone -broth-for-digestion-arthritis-and-cellulite/.

12. Ibid.

13. In e-mail conversation with author, June 15, 2016.

14. O'Connor, "Fasting Diets Are Gaining Acceptance."

15. Stephanie Bair, "Intermittent Fasting: Try This at Home for Brain Health," *Law and Sciences Blog*, January 9, 2015, accessed September 6, 2016, https://law .stanford.edu/2015/01/09/lawandbiosciences-2015-01-09-intermittent-fasting-try -this-at-home-for-brain-health/.

16. Jose Antonio, "Intermittent Eating," March 31, 2016, International Society of Sports Nutrition, accessed September 6, 2016, http://www.theissnscoop.com /intermittent-eating/.

17. Michael Mosley and Mimi Spencer, *The FastDiet* (New York: Simon and Schuster, 2015), 37.

18. O'Connor, "Fasting Diets Are Gaining Acceptance."

19. Ibid.

CHAPTER 3—WATER AND FASTING

1. Foster, "The Healing Power of Juicing."

2. Ibid.

3. "Water Fasting," All About Fasting.

4. Ibid.

5. F. Batmanghelidj, *Your Body's Many Cries for Water* (Vienna, VA: Global Health Solutions, Inc., 1997), 99.

6. Melina Jampolis, "Expert Q&A: Can Drinking Lots of Water Help You Lose Weight?," CNN.com, April 10, 2009, accessed September 6, 2016, http://www .cnn.com/2009/HEALTH/expert.q.a/04/10/water.losing.weight.jampolis/index .html.

7. M. Boschmann et al., "Water-Induced Thermogenesis," *Journal of Clinical Endocrinology and Metabolism* 88, no. 12 (December 2003): 6015–6019.

8. Melina Jampolis, "Expert Q&A: Can Drinking Lots of Water Help You Lose Weight?," CNN.com, April 10, 2009, accessed September 23, 2016, http://www.cnn.com/2009/HEALTH/expert.q.a/04/10/water.losing.weight.jampolis/index.html.

9. "Activity: Water and Electrostatic Forces," Exploring Our Fluid Earth, accessed September 6, 2016, https://manoa.hawaii.edu/exploringourfluidearth/chemical/properties-water/types-covalent-bonds-polar-and-nonpolar/activity-water-and-electrostatic-forces; Jonathan Eisen, "Fact Sheet: DNA-RNA-Protein," Microbiology of the Built Environment Network, accessed September 6, 2016, http://microbe.net/simple-guides/fact-sheet-dna-rna-protein/.

10. Joseph Mercola, "Bottled Water Poisons Your Body One Swallow at a Time," Mercola.com, January 15, 2011, accessed September 6, 2016, http://articles.mercola.com/sites/articles/archive/2011/01/15/dangers-of-drinking-water-from-a-plastic-bottle.aspx; Joseph Mercola, "Villages in India Show the U.S. Just How Dangerous Fluoride in Our Water Is…," Mercola.com, July 20, 2010, accessed September 6, 2016, http://articles.mercola.com/sites/articles/archive/2010/07/20/indian-children-blinded-crippled-by-fluoride-in-water.aspx.

11. Wendi Parrish, "Sun Charged Water: Sun Power," NaturalFeetFootzonology.com, accessed September 6, 2016, http://www.naturalfeetfootzonology.com/suns-power.html; Nancy Hearn, "Sunlight Nutrition: the Biological Benefits of Sunlight to Human Health," Water Benefits Health, accessed September 6, 2016, http://www.waterbenefitshealth.com/sunlight-nutrition.html.

12. Joseph Mercola with Rachael Droege, "Nuts About Coconuts: Everything You Need to Know About This Supreme Health Food," Mercola.com, March 10, 2004, accessed September 7, 2016, http://articles.mercola.com/sites/articles/archive/2004/03/10/coconuts.aspx.

13. Guy Fagherazzi et al., "Consumption of Artificially and Sugar-Sweetened Beverages and Incident Type 2 Diabetes in the Etude Epidémiologique auprés des femmes de la Mutuelle Générale de l'Education Nationale–European Prospective Investigation Into Cancer and Nutrition Cohort," *American Journal of Clinical Nutrition* 97, no. 3 (March 2013): 517–523.

14. Mark Hyman, "How Diet Soda Makes You Fat (and Other Food and Diet Industry Secrets)," *Huffington Post*, May 7, 2013, accessed September 7, 2016, http://www.huffingtonpost.com/dr-mark-hyman/diet-soda-health_b_2698494.html.

15. "Homeostasis: Kidneys and Water Balance, Association of the British Pharmaceutical Industry, accessed September 7, 2016, http://www.abpischools.org.uk/page/modules/homeostasis_kidneys/kidneys6.cfm.

CHAPTER 4—YOU NEED TO DETOX

1. Sara Goodman, "Tests Find More Than 200 Chemicals in Newborn Umbilical Cord Blood," *Scientific American*, December 2, 2009, accessed September 7, 2016, http://www.scientificamerican.com/article/newborn-babies-chemicals-exposure-bpa.

2. Children's Environmental Health Center, "Children and Toxic Chemicals," Mount Sinai Hospital, accessed September 7, 2016, http://www.mountsinai.org/patient -care/service-areas/children/areas-of-care/childrens-environmental-health-center /childrens-disease-and-the-environment/children-and-toxic-chemicals.
3. Victoria Colliver, "Toxics Found in Pregnant U.S. Women in UCSF Study," *SF Gate*, January 14, 2011, accessed September 7, 2016, http://www.sfgate.com /health/article/Toxics-found-in-pregnant-U-S-women-in-UCSF-study-2478903 .php.
4. Dr. Charles, *The Toxin Avoidance Handbook*, Perfect Origins, e-book, copyright © 2012, accessed September 7, 2016, http://www.perfectorigins.com/Toxin_ Avoidance.pdf.
5. Jeffrey Norris, "Chemicals in Environment Deserve Study for Possible Role in Fat Gain, Says Byers Award Recipient," University of California–San Francisco, News Center, December 15, 2010, accessed September 7, 2016, https://www.ucsf .edu/news/2010/12/6017/obesity-pesticides-pollutants-toxins-and-drugs-linked -studies-c-elegans.
6. Ibid.
7. Ibid.
8. Joseph Mercola, "Nine Health Risks That Aren't Worth Taking," Mercola.com, June 18, 2012, accessed September 7, 2016, http://articles.mercola.com/sites /articles/archive/2012/06/18/nine-health-risks-habits.aspx.

CHAPTER 5—THE DETOX FAST

1. David Williams, "Detox Naturally With Cilantro and Clay," DrDavidWilliams. com, August 5, 2015, accessed September 12, 2016, http://www.drdavidwilliams .com/cilantro-clay-for-detoxification/.
2. Ibid.
3. Ibid.

CHAPTER 6—FREQUENTLY ASKED QUESTIONS ABOUT FASTING

1. Judy Siegel-Itzkovich, "Doctors: Fasting During All but Last Weeks of Pregnancy Increases Risks," *Jerusalem Post*, September 11, 2013, accessed September 13, 2016, http://www.jpost.com/Health-and-Science/Doctors-Fasting-during-all-but -last-weeks-of-pregnancy-increases-risks-325894.
2. "Fasting in Pregnancy," BabyCentre, reviewed July 2013, accessed September 13, 2016, http://www.babycentre.co.uk/a1028954/fasting-in-pregnancy.
3. Chhandita Chakravarty, "Five Useful Tips to Make Fasting Easier While Breast-feeding," Mom Junction, June 13, 2016, accessed September 13, 2016, http:// www.momjunction.com/articles/tips-to-make-fasting-easier-while-breast-feeding_00119775.
4. Joseph Mercola, "Should You Eat Before Exercise?," Mercola.com, September 13, 2013, accessed September 13, 2016, http://fitness.mercola.com/sites/fitness /archive/2013/09/13/eating-before-exercise.aspx.
5. Ibid.

6. Kelly Turner, "Is It Healthy to Exercise While Fasting?," Fitday.com, accessed September 13, 2016, http://www.fitday.com/fitness-articles/fitness/exercises/is-it-healthy-to-exercise-while-fasting.html.

7. Renu Gandhi and Suzanne M. Snedeker, "Consumer Concerns About Pesticides in Food," Fact Sheet #24, Cornell University Program on Breast Cancer and Environmental Risk Factors in New York State, Cornell University, March 1999, accessed September 13, 2016, https://ecommons.cornell.edu/bitstream/handle/1813/14534/fs24.consumer.pdf.

8. L. Horrigan, R. S. Lawrence, and P. Walker, "How Sustainable Agriculture Can Address the Environmental and Human Health Harms of Industrial Agriculture," *Environmental Health Perspectives* 110, no. 5 (May 2002), as referenced in "Pesticides," Grace Communications Foundation, accessed September 13, 2016, http://www.sustainabletable.org/263/pesticides.

9. A. Ascherio et al., "Pesticide Exposure and Risk for Parkinson's Disease," *Annals of Neurology* 60, no. 2 (August 2006): 197–203.

10. L. A. McCauley et al., "Studying Health Outcomes in Farmworker Populations Exposed to Pesticides," *Environmental Health Perspectives* 114, no. 6 (June 2006): 953–960.

11. Maya Shetreat-Klein, *The Dirt Cure: Growing Healthy Kids With Food Straight From Soil* (New York: Simon and Schuster, 2016), 172.

12. Environmental Working Group, "Executive Summary: EWG's 2016 Shopper's Guide to Pesticides in Produce," accessed September 13, 2016, https://www.ewg.org/foodnews/summary.php.

13. Tara Parker-Pope, "Five Easy Ways to Go Organic," *Well* (blog), *New York Times*, October 22, 2007, accessed September 13, 2016, http://well.blogs.nytimes.com/2007/10/22/five-easy-ways-to-go-organic/.

14. "Shopper's Guide to Pesticides in Produce," Environmental Working Group, accessed September 13, 2016, https://tripinsurancestore.com/4/EWG_pesticide.pdf.

15. "Dirty Dozen," EWG's 2016 Shopper's Guide to Pesticides in Produce, accessed September 13, 2016, https://www.ewg.org/foodnews/dirty_dozen_list.php.

16. "Clean Fifteen," EWG's 2016 Shopper's Guide to Pesticides in Produce, accessed September 13, 2016, https://www.ewg.org/foodnews/clean_fifteen_list.php.

17. Ibid.

18. Foster, "The Healing Power of Juicing."

19. Ibid.

CHAPTER 7—THE QUICK AND EASY JUICE-FAST MENU AND RECIPES

1. Joseph Mercola, "Benefits of Beets," Mercola.com, January 25, 2014, accessed September 13, 2016, http://articles.mercola.com/sites/articles/archive/2014/01/25/beets-health-benefits.aspx.

2. "Cabbage: What's New and Beneficial About Cabbage," The World's Healthiest Foods, accessed September 13, 2016, http://www.whfoods.com/genpage.php?tname=foodspice&dbid=19.

3. Juliann Schaeffer, "Color Me Healthy—Eating for a Rainbow of Benefits," *Today's Dietitian*, November 2008, 34.

4. "What Is Spinach Good For?," Mercola.com, accessed September 13, 2016, http://foodfacts.mercola.com/spinach.html.

5. "Basil," The World's Healthiest Foods, accessed September 13, 2016, http://www.whfoods.com/genpage.php?tname=foodspice&dbid=85.

6. "Health Benefits of Carrots," Organic Facts, accessed September 13, 2016, https://www.organicfacts.net/health-benefits/vegetable/carrots.html.

7. C. D. Black et al., "Ginger (Zingiber Officinale) Reduces Muscle Pain Caused by Eccentric Exercise," *Journal of Pain* 11, no. 9 (September 2010): 894–903.

8. Bhrat B Aggarwal, Young-Joon Surh, Shishir Shishodia, eds., *The Molecular Targets and Therapeutic Uses of Curcumin in Health and Disease* (New York: Springer Science+Business Media, LLC, 2007), 360.

9. Judy Siegel, "Garlic Prevents Obesity," *Jerusalem Post*, October 30, 2001, 5.

10. Cherie Calbom, *The Juice Lady's Remedies for Diabetes* (Lake Mary, FL: Siloam, 2016), 27.

11. R. Alizadeh-Navaei, "Investigation of the Effect of Ginger on the Lipid Levels: A Double-Blind Controlled Clinical Trial," *Saudi Medical Journal* 29, no. 9 (September 2008): 1280–1284.

12. Nafiseh Khandouzi et al., "The Effects of Ginger on Fasting Blood Sugar, Hemoglobin A1c, Apolipoprotein B, Apolipoprotein A-1 and Malondialdehyde in Type 2 Diabetic Patients," *Iranian Journal of Pharmaceutical Research* 14, no. 1 (Winter 2015): 131–140.

13. Editors of Rodale Wellness, "Ten Foods That Can Lower Your Blood Sugar Naturally," *Prevention*, October 14, 2015, accessed September 13, 2016, http://www.prevention.com/food/foods-lower-blood-sugar.

14. R. D. Altman and K. C. Marcussen, "Effects of a Ginger Extract on Knee Pain in Patients With Osteoarthritis," *Arthritis and Rheumatism* 44, no. 11 (November 2001): 2531–2538.

15. "Cumin Seeds," The World's Healthiest Foods, accessed September 13, 2016, http://www.whfoods.com/genpage.php?tname=foodspice&dbid=91.

16. "Health Benefits of Zucchini," Organic Facts, accessed June 11, 2016, https://www.organicfacts.net/health-benefits/vegetable/health-benefits-of-zucchini.html.

CHAPTER 8—THE DANIEL FAST MENU PLAN

1. Adapted from Cherie Calbom, *The Juice Lady's Anti-Inflammation Diet* (Lake Mary, FL: Siloam, 2015), 78.

2. Ibid., 146.

3. "What Is Arugula Good For?," Mercola.com, accessed September 13, 2016, http://foodfacts.mercola.com/arugula.html.

4. Ibid.

5. Ibid.

6. "Squash, Summer," The World's Healthiest Foods, accessed September 13, 2016, http://www.whfoods.com/genpage.php?tname=foodspice&dbid=62.

7. Adapted from Calbom, *The Juice Lady's Anti-Inflammation Diet*, 117.

8. Ibid., 120–121.

9. "Tarragon (Artemisia Dracunculus)," HerbWisdom.com, accessed September 13, 2016, http://www.herbwisdom.com/herb-tarragon.html.

10. Cherie Calbom, "Broccoli to the Rescue!," accessed September 13, 2016, http://www.juiceladycherie.com/Juice/broccoli-to-the-rescue/.

11. "What Is Rhubarb Good For?," Mercola.com, accessed September 13, 2016, http://foodfacts.mercola.com/rhubarb.html.

12. "Eggplant," The World's Healthiest Foods, accessed September 13, 2016, http://www.whfoods.com/genpage.php?dbid=22&tname=foodspice.

13. Chris Obenschain, "Six Surprising Health Benefits of Pumpkins," CNN.com, October 21, 2014, accessed September 13, 2016, http://www.cnn.com/2014/10/21/health/health-benefits-of-pumpkin/.

14. Adapted from Calbom, *The Juice Lady's Anti-Inflammation Diet*, 109.

15. "Garbanzo Beans (Chickpeas)," The World's Healthiest Foods, accessed September 13, 2016, http://www.whfoods.com/genpage.php?tname=foodspice&dbid=58.

16. Adapted from Cherie Calbom, *The Juice Lady's Living Foods Revolution* (Lake Mary, FL: Siloam, 2011), 217.

17. Adapted from Cherie Calbom, *The Juice Lady's Turbo Diet* (Lake Mary, FL: Siloam, 2011), 195.

18. Ibid., 196.

19. Adapted from Cherie Calbom, *The Juice Lady's Sugar Knockout* (Lake Mary, FL: Siloam, 2016), 187.

CHAPTER 9—THE SPIRITUALITY OF FASTING

1. Marci Alborghetti, "Finding Rest: Keep It Holy, Saturday, April 16," in *Daily Guideposts 2016: A Spirit-Lifting Devotional* (Grand Rapids, MI: Zondervan, 2015), 117.

2. Abraham Joshua Heschel, *The Sabbath* (New York: Farrar, Straus and Giroux, 1951, 2005), 15.

3. David Brooks, "Why Is Clinton Disliked?," *New York Times*, May 24, 2016, accessed September 14, 2016, http://www.nytimes.com/2016/05/24/opinion/why-is-clinton-disliked.html.

4. Seewald, ed., *Wisdom From the Monastery*, 123–124.

5. *Merriam-Webster Online*, s.v. "driven," accessed September 14, 2016, http://www.merriam-webster.com/dictionary/driven.

6. David Fontes, *In the Eyes of Your Creator: Truly Valuing Yourself and Others* (Chesterton, IN: Ancient Faith Publishing, 2014), 33.

7. For a good discussion of the present implications of salvation, see N. T. Wright, *Surprised by Hope* (New York: HarperCollins, 2008).

8. Bernhard Müller, "Fasting in the Monastery," in Seewald, ed., *Wisdom From the Monastery*, 29.

9. Richard Foster, *Celebration of Discipline* (New York: HarperCollins, 1998), 55.

10. Susan Gregory, "The Daniel Fast," accessed September 14, 2016, http://daniel-fast .com/dont-settle-less-miss-best/.

11. John Piper, *A Hunger for God: Desiring God Through Fasting and Prayer* (Wheaton, IL: Crossway Books, 1997), 14.

12. James A. Kleist, trans., *The Didache*, Ancient Christian Writers Series, vol. 6 (New York: Paulist Press, 1948), 19.

13. Joan Brueggemann Rufe, as quoted in Kent D. Berghuis, *Christian Fasting: A Theological Approach* (Dallas: Biblical Studies Press, 2007), 77.

14. Clement of Alexandria, as quoted in Philip Schaff, *History of the Christian Church*, vol. 1: *From the Birth of Christ to the Reign of Constantine, AD 1–311* (New York: Charles Scribner and Company, 1870), 169.

15. For more information on the persecution of Christians and why they were perceived to be a threat, see Robin Phillips, *Saints and Scoundrels: From King Herod to Solzhenitsyn* (Moscow, ID: Canon Press, 2011), chapter 2.

16. *Ante-Nicene Fathers*, vol. 3, Allan Menzies, ed. *Latin Christianity: Its Founder, Tertullian*, chapter L, Christian Classics Ethereal Library, accessed September 14, 2016, http://www.ccel.org/ccel/schaff/anf03.iv.iii.l.html.

17. St. John Chrysostom, as quoted in Herbert Musurillo, "The Problem of Ascetical Fasting in the Greek Patristic Writers," *Traditio* 12 (1956): 59.

18. Herbert M. Shelton, *The Science and Fine Art of Fasting* (Chicago: Natural Hygiene Press, 1978), 137.

19. Cornelius Plantinga Jr., as quoted in Piper, *A Hunger for God*, 210.

20. Müller, "Fasting in the Monastery," in Seewald, ed., *Wisdom From the Monastery*, 16–17.

21. For a history of how monastic disciplines spread to the parish, see George E. Demacopoulos, *Five Models of Spiritual Direction in the Early Church* (Notre Dame, IN: University of Notre Dame Press, 2006).

22. Seewald, ed., *Wisdom From the Monastery*, 54.

23. Ron Lagerquist, "Ron Lagerquist's Fasting Testimony," FreedomYou.com, accessed September 14, 2016, http://www.freedomyou.com/ron_lagerquists_fasting_ testimony_freedomyou.aspx.

24. Ibid.

25. Ibid.

26. Seewald, ed., *Wisdom From the Monastery*, 59.

27. Otto Buchinger, as quoted in Seewald, ed., *Wisdom From the Monastery*, 75.

28. Foster, *Celebration of Discipline*, 55.

29. Isaac of Syria, as quoted in Richard Smoley, *Inner Christianity: A Guide to the Esoteric Tradition* (Boston: Shambhala, 2002), 62.

30. Müller, "Fasting in the Monastery," in Seewald, ed., *Wisdom From the Monastery*, 62.

31. Ibid.

32. Father Alexander Elchaninov, *The Diary of a Russian Priest* (Yonkers, NY: St. Vladimirs Seminary Press, 1997), as quoted in Mother Mary and Bishop Kallistos Ware, "The Meaning of the Great Fast: The True Nature of Fasting," Greek

Orthodox Archdiocese of America, accessed September 14, 2016, http://www .goarch.org/ourfaith/ourfaith9199.

33. Foster, *Celebration of Discipline*, 58–59.

34. Orthodox Church in America, "Lives of All Saints Commemorated on February 28," February 28, 2012, accessed September 14, 2016, https://oca.org/saints/all -lives/2012/02/28.

35. Philip Schaff and Henry Wace, eds., *A Select Library of Nicene and Post-Nicene Fathers of the Christian Church*, vol. 8, *St. Basil: Letters and Select Works* (New York: The Christian Literature Company, 1895), lxi.

36. St. Chrysostom, *The Homilies on the Statutes*, Homily III, in *St. Chrysostom: On the Priesthood; Ascetic Treatises; Select Homilies and Letters; Homilies on the Statutes*, Christian Classics Ethereal Library, accessed September 14, 2016, http:// www.ccel.org/ccel/schaff/npnf109.xix.v.html.

37. Mother Mary and Bishop Ware, "The Meaning of the Great Fast: The True Nature of Fasting."

Chapter 10—Fasting From Toxic Thinking and Emotions

1. Etty Hillesum, *Etty Hillesum* (New York: Henry Holt and Company, 1996), 144– 145.

2. Rebecca Ondov, "Saturday, April 23," in *Daily Guideposts 2016*, 124.

3. Barbara Hoberman Levine, *Your Body Believes Every Word You Say: The Language of Body/Mind Connection* (Fairfield, CT: WordsWork Press, 2000), book description on Barnes&Noble, accessed September 14, 2016, http://www.barnes andnoble.com/w/your-body-believes-every-word-you-say-barbara-hoberman-levine /1114299897.

4. Buryl Payne, as quoted in Levine, *Your Body Believes Every Word You Say*.

5. Stephan Rechtschaffen, foreword to *The Heartmath Solution* by Doc Childre and Howard Martin (New York: HarperCollins, 2000), ix.

6. Cherie Calbom and John Calbom, *The Complete Cancer Cleanse: A Proven Program to Detoxify and Renew Body, Mind, and Spirit* (Nashville: Thomas Nelson, 2006), 227.

7. Caroline Leaf, "You Are What You Think: 75–98% of Mental and Physical Illnesses Come From Our Thought Life!," DrLeaf.com, November 30, 2011, accessed September 14, 2016, http://drleaf.com/blog/you-are-what-you-think -75-98-of-mental-and-physical-illnesses-come-from-our-thought-life/.

8. Caroline Leaf, "C-Reactive Protein and How Our Bodies React to Toxic Thought," DrLeaf.com, June 1, 2015, accessed September 14, 2016, http://drleaf.com/blog /c-reactive-protein-and-how-our-bodies-react-to-toxic-thought/.

9. For research on how our thoughts affect our DNA, see Bret Stetka, "Changing Our DNA Through Mind Control?," *Scientific American*, December 16, 2014, accessed September 14, 2016, http://www.scientificamerican.com/article/ changing-our-dna-through-mind-control/; and HeartMath Institute, "You Can Change Your DNA," July 14, 2011, accessed September 14, 2016, https://www

.heartmath.org/articles-of-the-heart/personal-development/you-can-change-your
-dna/.

10. Caroline Leaf, "Thoughts Have a Viral Effect on Your Mind," DrLeaf.com, June
    27, 2011, accessed September 14, 2016, http://drleaf.com/blog/thoughts-have-a
    -viral-effect-on-your-mind/.

11. Caroline Leaf, *Switch On Your Brain: The Key to Peak Happiness, Thinking, and
    Health* (Grand Rapids, MI: Baker Books, 2013), 188.

12. Cherie Calbom with John Calbom, *Juicing, Fasting, and Detoxing for Life:
    Unleash the Healing Power of Fresh Juices and Cleansing Diets* (New York:
    Hachette Book Group, 2008), 237–238.

13. Robin Phillips, "How Peace of Mind Is a Skill That Can Be Developed With
    Practice," Taylor Study Methods, May 14, 2016, accessed September 15, 2016,
    http://www.taylorstudymethod.com/blog/how-to-develop-peace-of-mind/.

14. Ibid.

15. Ibid.

16. Ibid.

17. Ibid.

18. Ibid.

19. Ibid.

20. Ibid.

21. For an excellent overview of the science of neuroplasticity, see Norman Doidge,
    *The Brain That Changes Itself: Stories of Personal Triumph From the Frontiers of
    Brain Science* (New York: Penguin, 2007); and Norman Doidge, *The Brain's Way
    of Healing: Remarkable Discoveries and Recoveries From the Frontiers of Neuro-
    plasticity* (New York: Penguin, 2015).

22. Glen Rein and Rollin McCraty, "Local and Non-Local Effects of Coherent Heart
    Frequencies on Confrontational Changes of DNA," in *Proceedings of the Joint
    USPA/IAPR Psychotronics Conference*, Milwaukee, Wisconsin, 1993, accessed
    September 23, 2016, https://appreciativeinquiry.case.edu/uploads/Heart-
    Math%20article.pdf.

23. Richard H. Popkin, ed., *The Philosophy of the Sixteenth and Seventeenth Centuries*
    (New York: The Free Press, 1966), 14.

24. Matthias Forstmann, Pascal Burgmer, and Thomas Mussweiler, "'The Mind Is
    Willing, but the Flesh Is Weak': The Effects of Mind-Body Dualism on Health
    Behavior," *Psychological Science* 23, no. 10 (October 2012): 1239–1245.

25. Association for Psychological Science, "Mind vs. Body? Dualist Beliefs Linked
    With Less Concern for Healthy Behaviors," July 24, 2012, accessed September 15,
    2016, http://www.psychologicalscience.org/index.php/news/releases/mind-versus
    -body-dualist-beliefs-linked-with-less-concern-for-healthy-behaviors.html.

26. Shelton, *The Science and Fine Art of Fasting*, 137.

27. Rick Hanson, "Pay Attention," accessed September 15, 2016, http://www
    .rickhanson.net/pay-attention/.

28. Chade-Meng Tan, *Search Inside Yourself: The Unexpected Path to Achieving Suc-
    cess, Happiness (and World Peace)* (New York: HarperOne, 2014), as referenced

in Robin Phillips, "The Most Important 10 Minutes of Your Life," *UNpragmatic Thoughts* (blog), *Salvo*, July 7, 2016, accessed September 15, 2016, http://www.salvomag.com/unpragmatic-thoughts/?p=2621.

29. Leaf, *Switch On Your Brain*, 20.

30. Ibid., 72–73.

31. "The Heart-Brain Connection," HeartMath, accessed November 3, 2016, https://www.heartmath.org/programs/emwave-self-regulation-technology-theoretical-basis/.

32. "The Science Behind the emWave and Inner Balance Technologies," HeartMath, accessed September 15, 2016, http://www.heartmath.com/science-behind-emwave/. Used by permission granted on website.

33. These questions and the accompanying quotes come from workbook 1 in the Seven Areas of Life Training (SALT) series put out by Victorious Christian Living International.

34. Seven Areas of Life Training (SALT), vol. 1 (Goodyear, AZ: VCL International, 2006), 10.

35. Ibid.

36. Ibid.

37. Ibid., 12.

38. Ibid., 11.

39. Ibid., 13.

40. Ibid., 11–12.

41. Hale Dwoskin, *The Sedona Method Course Workbook: Your Key to Lasting Happiness, Success, Peace and Emotional Well-Being* (Sedona, AZ: Sedona Training Associates, 2000).

42. Karol K. Truman, *Feelings Buried Alive Never Die* (St George, UT: Olympus Distributing, 2003), 122.

APPENDIX—RESOURCES

1. "5 Tips to Be Your Own Heart Hero," HeartMath, accessed September 15, 2016, http://www.heartmath.com/blog/articles/5-tips-to-be-your-own-heart-hero/.

CONNECT WITH US!

CHARISMA HOUSE

(Spiritual Growth)

Facebook.com/CharismaHouse

@CharismaHouse

Instagram.com/CharismaHouseBooks

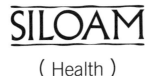

SILOAM

(Health)

Pinterest.com/CharismaHouse

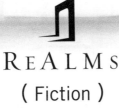

REALMS

(Fiction)

Facebook.com/RealmsFiction